NATURALLY ITALIAN

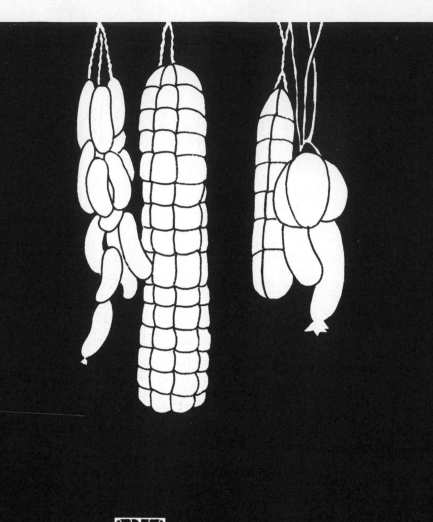

A Sunrise Book

E. P. DUTTON   •   NEW YORK

NATURALLY ITALIAN

A Treasury of Original Stay-Slim Italian Dishes
Prepared in Minutes

ELISA CELLI & INEZ M. KRECH

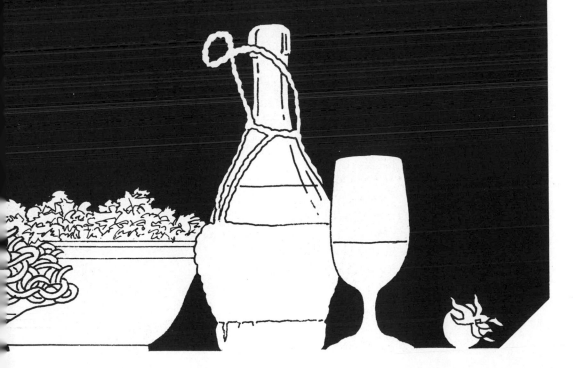

For information contact:
E. P. Dutton, 2 Park Avenue, New York, N.Y. 10016

Library of Congress Cataloging in Publication Data

Celli, Elisa.
Naturally Italian.

"A Sunrise book."
Includes index.
1. Low-calorie diet—Recipes.   2. Cookery, Italian.
I. Krech, Inez M., joint author.   II. Title.
RM222.2.C35   641.5'635   78–8162

ISBN: 0–87690–305–7

Published simultaneously in Canada by
Clarke, Irwin & Company Limited, Toronto and Vancouver

Designed by The Etheredges

10 9 8 7 6 5 4 3 2 1

First Edition

CONTENTS

---

* p. 62 - Chicken - NAPOLEON

PREFACE

If you had a childhood that exposed you to a great variety of delicious foods, you probably developed a knowledgeable palate. I had such a childhood. There were many special occasions as well as daily meals of beautifully prepared Italian dishes. My mother was and is an excellent cook with a great flair for presentation and creativity. She also loved to entertain, so we always had lots of guests for dinner. There was considerable emphasis on food in my family—the art of preparation, the joy of tasting well-prepared dishes, the wine, the fun and laughter of the varied occasions with relatives and friends.

My father owned a specialty Italian grocery store (Italian delicatessen, you might say), which provided another opportunity for learning. Not only did we see all sorts of food, often imported from Italy, but we also saw all sorts of people—a great educational experience. Exposure to good fresh food, well prepared, at a young age gives an understanding and a demanding palate that stays with us all our lives.

Being the only girl in a family with three brothers, I started at the age of seven to help my mother prepare the great Italian specialties for this or that *festa* as well as daily lunches and dinners. I remember the hours and days ahead of time my mother would spend preparing special dishes for a Sunday dinner or a weekday dinner for thirty people. And we always laughed because my mother used to say, "Oh, I am sorry, I didn't have much time to prepare something really special." Of course, everyone would reply, "What would you prepare if you did have time . . . this is *fantastico!*"

As soon as I could reach the top of the table I started to make the pasta that is a specialty of Pescara, in Abruzzi—*pasta alla chitarra.* Made on two boards strung with about ten guitar strings, the pasta dough is rolled over the guitar strings and falls through the spaces to the bottom, making the thinnest, greatest-tasting pasta. But, oh! how your arms hurt from pressing so hard over the guitar strings!

My father insisted on maintaining the same diet in America as in Italy, prepared as my mother learned in Pescara. Sometimes she had to use substitutes because she could not find the original ingredients here. When we returned to Italy for a visit and sampled the same dish, everyone would say *"Che sapore!"* which means "What taste!" or in effect, "That's the real taste!"

In order to reproduce that special savor, I hunted for products that tasted similar to those I remembered from Italy. Also, I wanted to cook in the same fashion as my mother did when entertaining friends, but it was difficult when I worked as an actress. After two years of experimenting I found a way to make these good things in minutes, and the results satisfied my mother and brothers, the hardest critics in the world. Everyone asked me for the techniques and recipes.

Most important, I began a sort of "crusade" to convince people that Italian food was not fattening. Americanized Italian food such as canned spaghetti, pizza, heavy sauces and fried foods can be fattening, but this was not the food I learned to prepare.

I found that lots of people shared these problems—no time for fussing but a great love for food and a wish to present it well. There was a need to prepare low-calorie meals; no chance to shop in obscure or fancy markets; a desire to eat more wholesome and natural foods.

I remember a special soup my mother made on Saturdays—*brodo con riso,* a chicken broth with rice and pieces of chicken and vegetables. I remember marvelous seafood; it was the main protein of our diet, since Pescara is on the Adriatic, surrounded by beautiful water on one side, with mountains on the other. I remember delicious vegetables. All these foods are part of this recipe collection; the emphasis on pasta, seafood, chicken and vegetables is personal, but the selection is also important for a nonfattening diet.

Some of the culinary treasures have been collected from the fourteen main regions of Italy and have never appeared, even in other versions, in any cookbook. The original recipes and adaptations were developed to be quick and easy to prepare, and light in calories. The recipes are based, as far as possible, on fresh natural ingredients. With few exceptions everything can be found in supermarkets, and the exceptions can be found in Italian groceries.

If you have tried all sorts of diets and found you missed really good food, try this style of quick cooking with little fat. These recipes make dishes that are neither boring nor bland, and they won't leave you feeling hungry.

Grazia multo! To all who have helped—first to my mother Adelaide D'Antonio. My brothers, Louis, Joseph and Robert. My editor, Pace Barnes; John Boswell our agent and special thanks to A. J. McClane and Inez Krech for her patience. My appreciation and thanks to Jimmy Cifu of Center Market for his splendid produce. And thanks to good friends, Ennio Riga, Leon Vogel, Sal Jamal, Dr. Peter Fodor, George Sojat, Hank Gruber, Deliah Henry, Glenn Moore, Honey Shun, Stella Arama, Enrico Serrante and Bruno Moschella.

New York   ELISA CELLI
February 1978

THE ITALIAN WAY

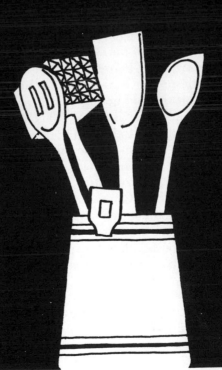

There is an authentic Italian way of life, a way of eating, a way of enjoying the gifts of nature. Italy is famous for its food, but the real thing, the natural food that is freshly prepared and served in an Italian home is different from the stereotype found in American-Italian restaurants or frozen and canned in markets. After years of trying to explain the difference, we have, in this book, made an effort to record the style of cooking used in Italian homes, converted for the American kitchen and using ingredients available in most supermarkets.

There are many Italian cookbooks—too many, you may believe. Often they are concerned with the rich diversity of regional cooking or with the elaborate food found in hotels and restaurants—the kind of food seen in Italian homes only on holiday occasions if at all. Some of these cookbooks are fine for reading, but when one looks at the number of ingredients and the amount of butter, cream and oil, the urge is to close the book. Such recipes are outdated in terms of today's needs when we have little time and still want to eat healthful foods and stay slim and attractive.

Italians put a great emphasis on the tradition of food, in preparation, taste, presentation and the "tradition of the meal." The main meal is in the middle of the day—*colazione,* from 12:00 to 3:00 P.M.—time for the family, an hour when everyone meets, shares, loves. It is healthier to have the main meal in the middle of the day; after lunch, Italian style, a brief rest period helps digestion. When you are relaxed, your metabolism works better and you burn food calories properly. The American style of eat and run with its accompanying tension plays a negative role in our attitudes about eating, in digestion, and in the process of burning up calories.

In Italy one can eat twice as much and not gain weight. This is because the food is fresh, natural, prepared carefully; it is light without grease, cream, refined sugar, preservatives and additives. Calories are reduced to begin with, but meals are balanced and presented in courses of small amounts. The style of service is more rigid in Italy than in other countries. When pasta is served, it is a first course, or main course in some special cases, but never a side dish. Meat is usually presented with only a side dish of vegetables. Quality is more important than quantity.

An Italian dinner is based on four or five courses: pasta; fish, poultry or meat, served with a vegetable accompaniment; salad; fruit and cheese; a sweet. A simpler menu would omit the sweet. There are regional differences; instead of pasta the first course might be *antipasto,* soup or risotto. For more elaborate occasions a simple *antipasto* such as prosciutto and melon may be served before the pasta.

This sample calorie-comparison chart shows the difference in calories between dishes prepared in the *Naturally Italian* method (without heavy oil, butter, cream, white flour, sugar) and the normal cooking method.

DINNER	CALORIES IN *Naturally Italian* METHOD	CALORIES IN NORMAL COOKING METHOD
Pasta Primavera	235	347
Chicken Sarna	210	605
Fennel and Rugola Salad	50	263
fresh strawberries (½ cup)	30	30
sauced with a few spoonfuls of Diana's Cold Zabaglione	90	120
wine: Pinot Grigio (white)	90 per glass	90
espresso coffee		
total calories	705	1455

DINNER	CALORIES IN *Naturally Italian* METHOD	CALORIES IN NORMAL COOKING METHOD
Fennel Soup	40	195
Veal Piccata alla Enrico	300	420
Italian Green Beans with Herbs	60	167
Watercress and Cucumber Salad	80	296
Ricotta Cheese Torta with Fruit	80	255
wine: Inferno (red)	100 per glass	100
espresso coffee		
total calories	660	1433

A luncheon or a supper will be simpler. For a buffet lunch (or brunch) several dishes will be prepared.

LUNCH	CALORIES IN *Naturally Italian* METHOD	CALORIES IN NORMAL COOKING METHOD
Risotto (with mixed seafood)	225	390
Fennel and Mushroom Salad	50	165
Grapefruit and Banana Ice alla Taormina	90	250
wine: Orvieto (white)	90 per glass	90
espresso coffee		
total calories	455	895

BUFFET LUNCH	CALORIES IN *Naturally Italian* METHOD	CALORIES IN NORMAL COOKING METHOD
Frittata (with vegetable filling)	135	235
with Tomato Sauce	80	100
Zucchini Misto	85	195
whole-wheat Italian bread or rolls	70	70
mixed fresh fruit with Grand Marnier	100	250
wine (choice): Corvo (white)		
Gattinara (red)	100 per glass	100
espresso coffee with cinnamon		
total calories	570	950

These menus are not intended to be a "starvation diet" but to be ample food for a normal person. If you think the calories are not low enough, you may be interested to learn that Chicken Sarna was developed from a chicken and mustard dish that had as many calories as the entire menu.

For informal occasions a one-dish meal may be served. Pasta dishes, especially lasagne and *timballo,* are good; also fish soups and stews, *risotto,* main-course *frittatas* and stuffed vegetables. All one-dish recipes are listed in the index.

Italy has been unified as one political entity only since 1871. Until then it was divided into a collection of small principalities and religious states. The mountainous country with practically no connecting roads (except the old Roman roads, which still exist) prevented the flow of goods and intercommunication among people. Political and geographical isolation, customs barriers, natural distrust of strangers, all contributed to the development of separate regional dialects and separate regional cuisines. In each area the ingredients at hand were used—fish and seafood on the coast; cornmeal in the extreme North; rice in the valleys of northern rivers; flour in the South; beef where there was grazing; veal where there was less pasture; pork and lamb where grazing was minimal. Even though a recipe name may seem classic or standard, in each region it might result in a different-tasting dish. For instance a seafood dish from Pescara, on the Adriatic, may be prepared with wine, lemon and herbs, while the same seafood prepared in Naples, on the Tyrrhenian Sea, will be cooked with tomatoes, garlic and olives. It is not only the local supplies but also the temperament of the area.

In this book you may read some classic names and be surprised at the ingredients or methods on the page. It may be that your version came from another region. In *Naturally Italian* the recipes have been recast to make them less fattening. The ingredients are faithful to the original, but there may be less of some of them. Fat, butter, cream, flour add texture to a dish, but basically not flavors, so we may use less of some of these, or none. But herbs and spices are taste accenters, and more may be added to make the dishes tastier.

In Italian homes where economy was a necessity, every scrap of food had to provide maximum nutrition. The low-fat natural dishes in this book are similar to those, with an emphasis on good nutrition. When there was no refrigeration, daily shopping was essential. While we can't suggest that, we do at least propose fresh ingredients, not packaged, canned, frozen. The true Italian taste comes from the natural taste of the basic ingredients—fresh fish, veal, vegetables, herbs—prominent in the dish, not camouflaged by heavy sauces or thickeners.

Any true gourmet cook must experiment with foods until the taste is just right. The artist comes alive in the experimental-creative stages of food preparation. Taste often as you cook and you will learn just what ingredient to use for a particular taste, and just what amount. When you have cooked following the methods described here, you'll discover that you can apply them to any other style of cooking and that you can adapt your old favorite recipes to be lower in calories and more nutritious; and you can create your own recipes using your family's preferred foods.

When you entertain, do you find yourself in the kitchen cooking and stirring while your guests enjoy the conviviality you are missing? The brief cooking time for these recipes will make it possible for you to share the pleasure with your guests. If you wish, you can sip your *aperitivo* between steps while they enjoy theirs.

The United States is the most-fed nation in the world, but it is becoming the worst-fed. We are eating more but being nourished less. Depleted soil, chemical fertilizers, food additives and preservatives, and poor eating habits are basic reasons, but destructive cooking methods are also to blame. Packaged and already prepared foods, so-called convenience foods, have all sorts of chemicals added to prevent mold and rancidity and to allow for longer shelf life. There are bleaches and dyes used to keep natural color, or maybe to make the food more colorful than it was. There are emulsifiers, antisprouting agents.

The point of this book, therefore, is to encourage you to change your whole approach to food—how you choose it and buy it as well as how you cook it and serve it. It's not a diet cookbook. It's a style of eating that is a way of life.

In spite of the importance of business or job in American life, our true lives revolve around social and family occasions. To cook well and eat well requires love. A happy host is one who enjoys the marketing, preparation, cooking and also the anticipation of sharing. Texture, color, smell and taste are all very sensual. The preparation methods that preserve these intrinsic qualities in food will give you nourishing meals that are also delicious and beautiful. Every meal will be a joy for family and guests, and besides they'll all stay thin.

ITALIAN METHODS FOR ITALIAN MEALS

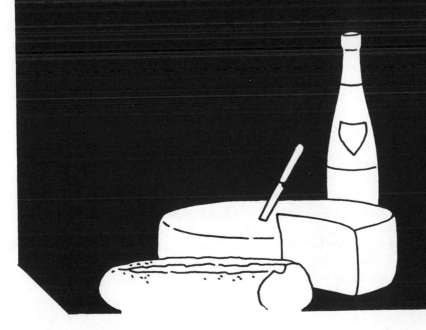

CHOOSING THE RIGHT INGREDIENTS

It is important to be selective with each ingredient you use in preparing a dish. Classic Italian food is based on the finest ingredients in food and wine, from the simplest tidbit to the most elaborate dessert. There are still various regional styles of cooking rather than a single Italian cuisine because it is considered sensible to make use of the produce at hand, special to the region or locality, and to buy it at the peak of ripeness (vegetables, fruits) or at the best season (fish, shellfish). The American style of selling hothouse asparagus or tomatoes or strawberries all year long is not followed in Italy. Even cheese is seasonal, as it is produced when the milk is richest.

Italians use the aromatics that grow in abundance on the hillsides and in the valleys of Italy—basil, rosemary, garlic, fennel. Olive oil and wine, produced since the days of the early Roman Empire, are basic to this cuisine, and delicious vegetables and fruits are Italian specialties. Unfortunately we cannot find exactly the same ingredients in our markets. Even our own fresh seasonal produce will taste different because of the differences in climate and soil. Processed foods from Italy available in American markets may be as close as you can get to the real Italian flavors, but they will also be different from the fresh foods before processing.

BUTTER: Butter is seldom used in these recipes, but when it is, unsalted butter is specified. Some dishes need the flavor of butter rather than oil. Unsalted butter does not keep for months, as salted butter does; this fresher butter has a more delicate taste, and the less salt the better. Do not use margarine. One tablespoon of butter contributes only 100 calories, actually less than 1 tablespoon of oil, but it is a saturated fat, therefore not recommended for low-cholesterol diets. It burns more quickly than oil, so it is inadvisable to use butter alone for high-heat sautéing. Butter can be used when sautéing over low heat, but oil should be added to it for high heat. For most sautéing oil is recommended, which see.

CHEESE: Italy makes lots of delicious cheeses, but not all are exported to America. Gorgonzola, Fontina, Bel Paese, Provolone, Taleggio, Parmesan and pecorino are imported. *Gorgonzola* is one of the great cheeses of the world, a mold-ripened blue cheese (although it looks green rather than blue), with a buttery texture. *Fontina* and *Bel Paese,* medium-soft ivory-colored cheeses, are excellent accompaniments to fruit; *Fontina* is especially good for melted cheese dishes. *Provolone,* a semihard cheese shaped by hand into rounds or shapes of melons, sausages or pears, is usually tied with strings; it can be natural or smoked. *Taleggio* is soft and creamy, like an immature Camembert. *Parmesan* and *pecorino* are hard cheeses, used for grating.

Parmesan, the best-known grating cheese in America, is exported from Italy only after aging for two years. For a delicious alternate, look for pecorino, made of sheep's milk. The most familiar type of pecorino in America is Romano, a pungent strong cheese in Italy, but here generally mild and much less flavorful than Parmesan. All pecorino cheeses are not Romano; Italian markets carry more pungent types. Both of these cheeses are high in calories, but they are so flavorful only a little is needed. The best you can buy is the best buy. Now, don't spoil the whole dish by buying it already grated, whether in a jar or carton! Not only is this less flavorful, it is also far more expensive. Grate only when you are ready to use it!

Ricotta, a cheese originally made from whey, is produced in the United States, and is now made of whey and milk, whole milk, skim milk or part-skim milk. Ricotta looks much like cottage cheese; if you need a substitute, skim-milk cottage cheese has the same calorie count as skim-milk ricotta. Ricotta is sweeter-tasting than cottage cheese; it is also more perishable; buy it fresh and use it promptly; most cartons today are dated. In Italy ricotta is made without salt; here most kinds have some salt. In recipes using ricotta we have found very little difference in flavor between a dish made with whole-milk cheese and the same dish made with skim-milk cheese. Skim-milk ricotta is recommended, but if you can find only "part-skim" use it instead; it is more generally available.

Mozzarella is made of whole milk, skim milk and part-skim. Again, use part-skim if you cannot find skim-milk mozzarella. Part-skim cheese has about one-fourth less calories than the same weight of whole-milk mozzarella. *Provatura* is mozzarella made of buffalo milk, shaped in smaller rounds than other cheese of this type in Italy or America. It is not easy to find this in America, but some Italian markets will have *mozzarella in buffo*—the little cheeses in water. Whether made of cow's milk or buffalo's milk, this snow-white cheese is light, easy to digest, bland-tasting; it can be cut (the name means "cheese that can be cut") or shredded easily and is perfect for melting. If you are lucky you may find a shop that has fresh mozzarella, which is more delicious than the usual plastic-wrapped cheeses.

Richer cheeses such as Gorgonzola or *ricotta salata,* a pressed and salted version, are used in small amounts only.

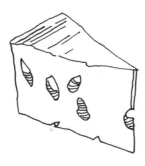

CREAM: Cream is used very seldom. If you love the taste and texture of creamy dishes, here are two ideas. Whip evaporated skim milk to replace cream, or use whipped ricotta cheese instead.

FISH: Use fresh fish and buy it in a responsible market you can depend on. A fresh fish has red gills, clear eyes, firm texture and no objectionable odor. Fresh does not mean "recently defrosted"; a good market will label fish so you can choose with confidence.

Clams, oysters and mussels should be alive, with shells tightly closed. A fresh lobster should be lively. A few exceptions: Spiny lobster *(aragosta)* and lobsterettes *(scampi)* are not found fresh in northern markets; they are available frozen. Canned anchovy fillets, in small amounts, are used for flavor accents, and there is one recipe for salt cod.

Plan to use fish or shellfish the day you buy it; every day seafood is out of the water it loses flavor.

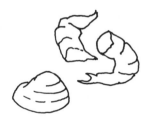

FLOUR: As much as possible avoid white flour and foods made with white flour. Whole-wheat flour and all-purpose flour, whether regular or enriched, have the same calories per volume, but the nutritional value of whole-wheat flour is greater; it has more protein, calcium and B vitamins.

FRUIT: It's tempting to say "always fresh," but fruits are not always available fresh, or they are pallid hothouse specimens or tasteless cold-storage produce. As a second choice use frozen fruits, but avoid canned. Some dried fruits are used, especially raisins, but these are extremely high in concentrated natural sweetness, so extremely high in calories; use only small amounts.

Fruits are often used as part of an *antipasto* selection, and they make a perfect close to a meal. Small amounts of fresh and dried fruits are added to fish and meat dishes to give a touch of natural sweetness. They are good additions to salads.

An exception: pineapple canned in its own natural juices can substitute for fresh when pineapples are not in season.

GARLIC: A favorite Italian flavoring. Buy plump heads with shiny cloves. Store in the refrigerator so it does not dry out. Most recipes use garlic puréed through a press; this flavors the dish more evenly and no one will have any pieces to bite on. The bugaboo of garlic breath is avoided this way. Some recipes use peeled whole cloves to flavor oil, then discard the cloves; another way to flavor a dish without risking garlic breath. Use for accenting sauces and dressings, vegetables, soups.

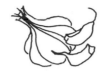

HERBS: These are primary flavorings for Italian dishes. If you can get them fresh, do so. Herbs can be raised in home gardens if there is adequate sun, even in pots in kitchen windows. If you harvest or buy more than you can use, freeze them in plastic or foil packets, or store them in a jar, with oil brushed on both sides of the leaves, in the refrigerator. If fresh is unavailable, use dried whole herbs. Ground herbs have usually lost most of their flavor by the time you buy them. Replace your packets of dried herbs every three months; they lose flavor and when too old add a dry texture to the dish.

Italian seasoning is used often in these recipes; this is a dried herb mixture, usually consisting of orégano, basil, rosemary, sage and savory. Some recipes include marjoram and thyme as well. Taste the mixture if you can before buying, because some have so much orégano that one can scarcely taste anything else.

Chives are available frozen in most supermarkets. Other herbs hard to find fresh are dill, rosemary, tarragon and thyme. Basil is available fresh only in the summer or early fall. Bay leaf and fennel seed are usually found only in dried form.

Parsley is for sale fresh all year long. Fresh parsley is useful in herb mixtures to counteract the dry taste of other dried herbs. In this book "Italian parsley" is specified throughout. That's not chauvinism rampant; this is a different kind of parsley. It has a somewhat coarser look, with flatter, less curly leaves; it is often labeled "flat-leaf parsley" and is more flavorful than the other kind.

HOT TASTE: Use cayenne pepper, crushed red pepper, curry powder, Tabasco or various chili peppers. Fresh gingerroot is also a good choice.

LEMON JUICE: A great flavor accent that brings out the tastes of the other ingredients. Italians use lemon juice on every type of food—chicken, lamb, veal, fish, vegetables, salads, appetizers, desserts. When possible, replace vinegar with lemon juice; it will add vitamin C. One tablespoon lemon juice will add 5 calories but contribute 7 milligrams of vitamin C. Squeeze lemon juice only just before using it; otherwise vitamin C is lost through oxidation. Lemon rind is also a good addition, since it has the aromatic lemon oil which carries the intense lemon flavor. Lemon juice is less acid than vinegar but more acid than other citrus juices or wine.

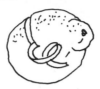

MEATS: The lack of fuel for cooking in Italy has limited meat cookery for the most part to small thin portions that can be cooked quickly; typical is the *scaloppina,* a slice cut from the leg of veal. Also, large pieces of meat for roasting, common in some other cuisines, need natural internal fat or larding or barding, since roasting is a dry cooking method. Roasts like this are high in calories.

Veal, lamb and chicken are the preferred meats in Italian cuisine. They are lighter, more digestible and less caloric than beef and pork. Veal and chicken have a similar delicacy of taste, and most recipes for one can be adapted for the other. (Many preparations can be used for fish, since it is also light, with delicate taste.)

Beef has been treated with all sorts of chemicals and hormones in an effort to make it tender, which makes it suspect from a health standpoint. Since lamb and veal are young animals, they have not been treated with additives; their young age makes them naturally tender. Also, the well-marbled American beefsteak is tremendously high in calories. There are recipes for beef in this book, but none for pork. Pork is too fatty for thin cooking. Ham, prosciutto (dry-cured Italian ham) and bacon are used occasionally but in small amounts, for taste accents.

MUSTARD: Usually prepared Dijon mustard is used, occasionally dry mustard. The natural mustard taste is present in these, whereas those prepared mustards with additional spices give quite a different flavor accent. Mustard is thought of as a "hot" accent, but it is actually very mild when added to recipes.

OIL: Olive oil contributes a specific delicious taste. When this is important, it is preferred to other oils. It has an important disadvantage—it is monounsaturated, therefore less useful for low-cholesterol diets than the polyunsaturated oils such as corn, safflower, sesame, etc. We like one specific oil—Wesson Oil, made of soybean and cottonseed; it is high in polyunsaturated fatty acids and contains no cholesterol. It is light and does not affect the flavor of other ingredients. One tablespoon contributes 120 calories, 10 less than the same amount of olive oil.

OLIVES: Yes, these have lots of calories, but they are so delicious and flavorful that only a few can add a lot to a dish. There are many olives other than brine-packed green or black; some are used in the recipes.

ONIONS: Other than garlic (a member of the onion family), the most often used onion is the shallot. Shallots grow like garlic, in a cluster with many little cloves or bulblets, each encased in a red skin. The flavor is intense but delicate. Also white onions, yellow onions, and large slicing onions are used.

PASTA: Many American brands of pasta are made with durum semolina, but none is the equal of imported Italian pasta. The recommended brand is Pastificio del Verde, Fara San Martino. All pasta made with durum semolina has a similar calorie count (210 calories per 2 ounces of uncooked pasta), but they are not all equally nutritious or delicious. You will find regular pasta, spinach pasta including spinach spaghetti, and tomato pasta, and in all the usual shapes and forms.

In Italy pasta is eaten every day, but it is served with delicate sauces, chiefly based on vegetables. Pasta is a separate course usually, and only small amounts are presented.

RICE: The round-grained rice from Piedmont, Arborio rice, is the most delicious rice for all Italian rice dishes. However, it isn't available everywhere. Instead use natural brown rice, which is more nutritious than polished rice, since it still has the whole grain, or use Carolina long-grain rice. Any of these is preferred to pretreated, precooked or processed rice. Brown rice is slightly more caloric than polished rice, but the added nutritive values more than outweigh this.

SALT: Use sparingly. Vegetables have natural salt, and all meats and animal products including milk and cheese also have natural salt. We have mostly left the amount of salt to your discretion; just remember that salt added early becomes concentrated as cooking continues. One can always add more, but it is impossible to take it out. Most directions for cooking pasta direct the cook to use 2 tablespoons salt for 1 pound pasta. In our recipes we have used only 1 tablespoon salt for 1 pound pasta. You may omit salt if you prefer, or increase to taste.

Sea salt is just as salty as any other salt, but it does not contain various additives designed to make the salt flow easily. Use it if you prefer. If true salt is not allowed on your diet, there are herb flavorings, called "herb salts," which can be used, but most chemical salt substitutes taste so horrible that you would be better off cultivating a liking for no salt at all.

SPICES: Ground spices, like ground herbs, lose their flavor quickly. Try to use whole spices and crush or grind them just before using. To save space we have not said "freshly ground" each time we mention black pepper, but we recommend that you grind peppercorns just before use.

White pepper, dry mustard, nutmeg, allspice, coriander, etc., are available whole. With the exception of nutmeg, these spices can be crushed in a mortar or ground in a spice grinder. Nutmeg needs a grater, but it can be a simple device. Cinnamon is so difficult to grind that it's better to buy it already processed.

Fresh gingerroot is more pungent and delicious than ground ginger. If you buy more than you use at once, freeze the root, or peel it, cover with dry Marsala, and store in the refrigerator.

SUGAR: Avoid white sugar as much as possible, not because it is so caloric—it is less so than honey—but because it has nothing to offer but calories. Honey has some vitamins as well. Liqueurs are used to sweeten desserts because a sweet taste with a flavor accent is preferred. Good choices are sweet Marsala wine, Amaretto liqueur and Grand Marnier liqueur.

Fruits have natural sugar and so do most vegetables. Purées of fresh fruits often need no extra sugar but can be used as sweeteners, as can the even sweeter dried fruits.

TOMATOES: The best tomatoes for sauces are plum tomatoes, sometimes called "Italian tomatoes." They have firm texture which produces a good purée in cooking. Because of their shape and size, it is easy to split them and press out the seeds; seeds give bitterness to cooked dishes (although this happens with long cooking more than with the quick cooking of this book). Other tomatoes are used for stuffing, and they can be used for everything if you can't find plum tomatoes. Whether to peel or not depends on you for the most part. For some of the recipes the tomatoes need to be peeled, but if it doesn't say to do it, it isn't necessary; in fact the skins may add some flavor and texture.

When fresh tomatoes are out of season, canned peeled plum tomatoes make an excellent substitute in cooked dishes. They are especially convenient for winter saucemaking.

VEGETABLES: Use fresh vegetables! The difference they make in taste, appearance and nutrition is enormous. When a particular vegetable is out of season, why not use something else? Frozen vegetables are a second choice. Frozen artichoke hearts are convenient because we do not have any fresh artichokes as small as that. Except for tomatoes, canned vegetables are not recommended; they are too soft and have lost color and nutritive value.

A raw vegetable or salad should be served at every meal throughout the year. Raw foods contribute vitamins and minerals as well as bulk. Salads need not be elaborate, and they take little time in preparation. Vegetables are also excellent first courses; they will curb the appetite for larger portions of other foods and decrease the desire for sweets.

To prevent enzyme action, use only cold water to wash vegetables. Wash thoroughly, but do not soak them. Dry them, using a soft cloth for large specimens like eggplants and squashes, and shaking leafy ones in a salad dryer or rolling in a cloth towel. Store in plastic bags in the refrigerator. If you have a box with automatic defroster, it will have a noticeable drying effect on vegetables that are not wrapped. Even the crisper drawers will allow some moisture loss. Air and light pull out vitamin content too. Do not peel anything until you are ready to use it. For everyday use, buy fresh vegetables every three or four days.

For off-seasons, freeze your own produce. Wash and dry, then wrap in plastic bags or other freezer wrap in as whole a shape as possible. When solidly frozen, overwrap to prevent dehydration. Not all vegetables freeze well raw; you may need to blanch some of them.

WINE: Wine is a primary sauce blender, a taste accent, a digestive. White wines are good for delicate sauces, reds for heavier sauces, and Marsala, dry or sweet according to need, is an excellent flavor blender for main courses or desserts.

Wine contains two types of food elements, those providing energy and those providing nutrition. Wine has all thirteen of the minerals established as necessary to human life, as well as vitamins A, B, and C. Rich in vitamin B, the vitamin complex remains stable and does not deteriorate as wine ages. Grape sugars and the yeast that makes the wine contribute to the total nutritive value.

The alcohol and some of the calories are burned off in the cooking process, so wine in cooked dishes does not contribute to alcohol intake at all.

Don't believe that any old wine can be used in cooking. So-called cooking wines have such a bitter taste they actually detract rather than add to a dish. And if you read labels you will observe that these commercial cooking wines often have other ingredients, including salt, which can alter the whole taste balance. The wine you serve your guests is the wine you should use in cooking. The amount is usually small—¼ to 1 cup—but the taste must carry through; you should use the best wine you can afford. Fine Italian wines with their distinctive taste contribute to cooked dishes, and economically they are good value.

CALORIES

The calories listed with each recipe are based on USDA tables and were worked out as much as possible on the calories of each ingredient before cooking. There is some reduction through cooking, so this figure can be regarded as a potential rather than actual figure. Also, each ingredient you purchase may vary somewhat from the standard used in the tables because of the soil and climate where it was produced or, in the case of fish and meats, because of the way it was raised or fed, and there are seasonal variations as well.

IMPORTANT! The calorie figure has been worked out for the basic recipe. It will not apply if you prepare one of the variations or invent one of your own. See also calorie charts in Appendix I.

TIME

An experienced cook can prepare a five-course meal in minutes; a beginner will need longer. The figures listed are actual times used for preparation of the recipes, but you may need more minutes until you develop skill in the kitchen. One of the advantages of this cookery is quickness, which helps to keep the fresh taste as well as texture and nutritive content.

SERVINGS

The size of each portion is important. In the context of the whole meal, the servings indicated in this book are generous—enough to satisfy but not enough to stuff.

READING THE RECIPES

Please read the whole recipe, including variations, before you shop, and certainly before you start to prepare the ingredients for cooking. In this way you will be comfortable with the procedures; also, if you find an ingredient in the basic list that you don't have or don't care for, a glance at the variations may suggest an alternate.

Ingredients are listed as much as possible in the style of a shopping list. For instance, instead of calling for a volume of chopped tomatoes, we have given the weight of whole tomatoes, as they are purchased, and instead of calling for a cup measure of chopped mushrooms, we have given the weight of mushrooms you will need to buy. (This doesn't work for all ingredients; for instance, one buys a bunch of parsley but only a small part is needed for a recipe.) Our aim is to simplify marketing as much as possible.

EQUIPMENT

In spite of the current fascination with machines of all kinds, the recipes in this book can be prepared with few utensils, most of them quite simple. Here is a short list of necessary items:

one 8-quart pot with cover (for pasta and stock)
two saucepans, 1-quart and 2-quart size
two or three skillets or frying pans, preferably large
vegetable steamer
large colander
fine sieve or strainer
garlic press
food mill
electric blender. (This is the chief "machine" used in this cookery, and it is
    useful for everything from soups to desserts.)
pepper mill
spice grinder
whisks of several sizes
good knives, for chopping, carving, paring. (Be sure the knife you use most
    is a "perfect small knife" for you, which fits your hand comfortably.)
wooden spoons and/or paddles
skimmer
melon-ball scoop
copper bowl (if you beat egg whites)
baking pans (lined with nonstick coating)

A FEW COOKING TRICKS

•Soaking or boiling vegetables is the greatest culinary crime. This results in a 50 to 90 percent loss of taste and nutrition. Better methods are steaming for 4 to 8 minutes (according to the vegetable and how it is cut) and oil-steaming. For oil-steaming, heat 2 tablespoons oil in a heavy pan, add vegetables, and cover. Sauté and steam for 4 or 5 minutes. Another excellent method for vegetables is to simmer them in a small amount of milk; cover tightly and simmer for 4 minutes. Any milk remaining is used for saucing. There is no vitamin loss, and vegetables are milder and sweeter.

•To cut down on the amount of cooking oil, use a heavy skillet and heat it so that even a small amount of oil will quickly spread to cover the entire surface. Or use skillets with nonstick coating. Use oils that do not congeal at room temperature. Olive oil is used for flavor in some recipes, but unsaturated oils are used most often.

•One way to save time in cooking is to limit the number of utensils and steps. Most recipes require only one skillet. Everything put into the skillet is served in the completed dish, and therefore no food nutrients are lost. To save time in preparation, most vegetables and herbs are cut directly into the cooking pot. Peel or trim the garlic, shallots, onions, tomatoes, and chop them into the skillet when needed. A wrist action is used. Either hold the shallot still and with the other hand cut it, or hold the knife rigid and push the shallot against the blade, turning the vegetable until it is all chopped. If this is difficult for you, chop the ingredients on a sturdy chopping board with a sturdy chef's knife.

•Never follow cookbook recipes to the letter—this cookbook or any other—except in special baking recipes. Cook to your own taste! Experiment by substituting ingredients you like, or adding them. Try a chicken recipe for fish or veal, or a vegetable preparation for another vegetable. Many of the recipes are followed by variations. Try these, or invent your own.

•All stoves have quirks. Yours may be hotter or cooler than the stove used to prepare these recipes. Make a few tests with your stove and oven. If the recipe needs longer to be fully cooked, your temperature control may be at a lower level than the test stove. You can adjust your times accordingly.

ITALIAN WINES
FOR
ITALIAN FOOD

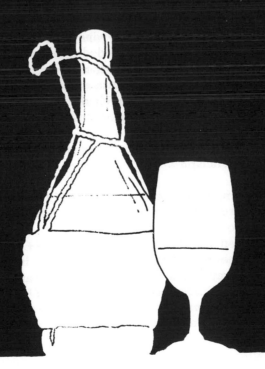

The list that follows is by no means a complete tally of Italian wines, but it will suggest the enormous variety to choose from. Many of the names will be new to you, since they are only now being imported. Ask your wine dealer to stock those that interest you; you will be pleasantly surprised by both quality and price.

PIEDMONT (PIEMONTE) and VALLE D'AOSTA: Asti Spumante *(sparkling white)*, Barbaresco *(red)*, Barolo *(red)*, Gancia *(sparkling white)*, Gattinara *(red)*, Ghemme *(red)*, Nebbiolo Piemontese *(red)*.

LIGURIA: Barbarossa *(red)*, Cinqueterre *(white)*, Vezzano *(red)*.

LOMBARDY (LOMBARDIA): Barbera *(red)*, Franciacorta *(white, red)*, Frecciarossa *(white, red, rosé)*, Grumello *(red)*, Inferno *(red)*, Nebbiolo *(red)*, Riesling (white), Sassella *(red)*.

VENETO: Bardolino *(red)*, Cabernet-Merlot *(red)*, Chianti *(red)*, Prosecco *(red)*, Raboso *(red)*, Recioto *(white)*, Recioto Soave *(white)*, Soave *(white)*, Tocai *(white)*, Valpolicella *(red)*.

TRENTINO–ALTO ADIGE: Cabernet *(red)*, Merlot *(red)*, Pinot Grigio *(white)*, Riesling *(white)*, Vino Santo *(sweet fortified)*.

FRIULI–VENEZIA GIULIA: Gamay *(red)*, Riesling *(white)*, Sauvignon *(red)*, Tocai *(white)*.

EMILIA-ROMAGNA: Albana *(white)*, Barbera *(red)*, Lambrusco *(red)*, Trebbiano *(white)*.

TUSCANY (TOSCANA): Brolio Riserva *(red)*, Brunello di Montalcino *(red)*, Chianti *(red)*, Chianti Classico *(red)*, Montecarlo *(white, red)*, Nipozzano *(red)*, Riserva Ducale *(aged red)*, Trebbiano Toscano *(white)*, Vernaccia di San Gimignano *(white)*, Villa Antinori *(red)*, Vino Nobile di Montepulciano *(red)*, Vino Santo *(sweet fortified)*.

UMBRIA: Nebbiolo *(red)*, Orvieto *(white)*, Trebbiano Spoletino *(white)*.

LATIUM (LAZIO): Castelli Romani *(white)*, Cori *(white, red)*, Est! Est! Est! di Montefiascone *(white)*, Frascati *(white)*.

MARCHES (MARCHE): Montepulciano del Conero *(red)*, Montesanto Rosso *(red)*, Verdicchio dei Castelli di Jesi *(white)*, Vino Santo *(sweet fortified)*.

ABRUZZO-MOLISE: Abruzzo Bianco or Trebbiano *(white)*, Abruzzo Rosso or Montepulciano *(red)*, Cerasuolo *(light red)*, Giulianova Bianco *(white)*, Peligno Bianco *(white)*.

Aosta

VALLE D'AOSTA

Milan

Bolzano

Trento

TRENTINO ALTO ADIGE

FRIULI-VENEZIA GIULIA

Turin

PIEDMONT

LOMBARDY

Udine

VENETO

Trieste

LIGURIA

EMILIA-ROMAGNA

Venice

Genoa

Bologna

Florence

TUSCANY

MARCHES

Ancona

Perugia

LATIUM

ABRUZZO

L'Aquila

Rome

Compobasso

MOLISE

Naples

CAMPANIA

APULIA

Bari

SARDINIA

Potenza

BASILICATA

Cagliari

CALABRIA

THE WINE PRODUCING REGIONS OF ITALY

Palermo

SICILY

Reggio di Calabria

CAMPANIA: Greco di Tufo *(white)*, Ischia Bianco *(white)*, Ischia Bianco Superiore *(white)*, Ischia Rosso *(red)*, Solopaca *(red)*.

APULIA (PUGLIA): Aleatico di Puglia *(light red)*, Castel del Monte *(white, red, rosé)*, Ostuni Bianco *(white)*.

CALABRIA: Ciro' *(white, red, rosé)*, Donnici *(red)*, Lametino *(red)*, Rubino *(red)*, Savuto *(red)*.

SICILY (SICILIA): Bianco Alcamo *(white)*, Cerasuolo di Vittoria *(red)*, Corvo *(white, red)*, Etna *(white, red, rosé)*, Malvasia delle Lipari *(sweet fortified)*, Marsala *(fortified, dry and sweet)*, Regaleali *(white, red)*, Segesta *(white, red)*.

SARDINIA (SARDEGNA): Cannonau di Sardegna *(red)*, Monica di Cagliari *(red)*, Vernaccia di Oristano *(white)*.

The table that follows will help you to choose wine of a type that best suits your menu.

WHITE WINES	
TYPES	VARIETIES
Mellow whites	Frascati abboccato
	Orvieto abboccato
	Prosecco
	Recioto Soave
	Vernaccia di San Gimignano
Dry, light-bodied whites	Corvo Bianco
	Est! Est! Est!
	Frascati Secco
	Pinot Grigio
Dry, medium-bodied whites	Orvieto Secco
	Soave
	Tocai
	Trebbiano
	Verdicchio
RED WINES	
TYPES	VARIETIES
Semidry reds	Lambrusco
Dry, light-bodied reds	Bardolino
	Cerasuolo

RED WINES

TYPES	VARIETIES
Dry, medium-bodied reds	Cabernet
	Chianti
	Grumello
	Inferno
	Montepulciano d'Abruzzo
	Merlot
	Nebbiolo
	Sassella
	Valpolicella
Robust reds	Barolo
	Barbaresco
	Brunello di Montalcino
	Chianti Riserva
	Corvo Rosso
	Gattinara
	Ghemme
	Vino Nobile di Montepulciano

ROSÉ, DESSERT AND SPARKLING WINES

TYPES	VARIETIES
Rosé wines	Castel del Monte
	Chiaretto
	Marino Rosé
Dessert wines	Marsala
	Vino Santo
Sparkling wines	Asti Spumante
	Gancia
	Nebbiolo Spumante
	Prosecco Spumante

WINE WITH FOOD

It is beyond doubt that one kind of wine is more pleasing to one palate and another to another, and that out of the winepress one wine will prove of outstanding excellence and far superior in breed to another either through the influence of the bottle or by chance. Wherefore each wine lover will depend on his own judgment as to the primacy of wines.

—PLINY THE ELDER (A.D. 23–79)

The marriage between food and wine can be one of the great pleasures of life if the complementary flavors are brought together properly. The combination can provide a taste satisfaction greater than food or wine could provide alone. The flavor and aroma of wine enhances the taste of food. Wine induces a sense of well-being, stimulates the taste buds, and relaxes the body to help digestion. Since the days of antiquity the dinner table has been an ideal setting for good food, good wine and good talk.

Wine should be preceded and followed by the products of the grape, not of the grain; wine and spirits do not go well together, and the mixture can spoil the taste of good food. Italians drink little hard liquor. However, at any hour during the day they may pause for an *aperitivo* such as vermouth, white or red, Martini or Cinzano, with or without *ghiaccio* (ice cubes). As to ice, there is an important and popular expression: "It is healthier to take drinks without ice." Herb-flavored drinks such as Campari, Cynar or Aperpol are good *aperitivos;* they relax the stomach but do not dull the taste buds. For the cook and hostess, who has spent time and care preparing a dinner, it is discouraging to have guests whose intake of hard liquor has numbed their sense of smell and taste so that they miss all the beauty of the food. Fortunately there is now a trend toward lighter drinks before lunch and dinner. Dry white wines or aromatized wines are being served more and more, with dry white wine the most popular apéritif. If this is your preference, choose a good Italian white—Corvo, Frascati, Orvieto, Pinot Grigio, Verdicchio, Vernaccia.

Wine rules have become less rigid, and choice is nowadays left to individual taste. The keener your taste, the better the choice. However, one must consider that the purpose of the wine is more than quenching the thirst; it must serve to enhance and complement the foods with which it is served. The following suggestions are a few simple basics for choosing wine to be served with food.

White wines go best with light foods such as appetizers, light first courses, fish, white meats, and pasta or risotto with light or creamy sauces. With a delicate dish serve a delicate wine. Red wines, which are stronger and heavier in taste, are usually served with hearty soups or stews, red meats, and pasta or risotto with heavy sauces. Look at the ingredients of the sauces to be served; coordinate the sauce taste with the wine, and if possible serve your guests the same wine used in the sauce. If you are in doubt as to the right choice, here is a good general rule: It is always safe to start with a dry white wine and to serve it throughout the meal. If you plan to serve two wines, start with the lighter white wine and serve the heavier red with a main course of beef, lamb or veal, or with a pasta dish of more substance sauced with meat or eggplant, or with a dish of baked lasagne.

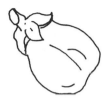

Some foods clash with wine, for instance, curries, spicy dishes and preparations made with vinegar. These can numb the taste buds and change the perception of the wine taste. A great dish needs a great wine to set it off; in contrast a fine wine can be "killed" when served with a poorly prepared dish or one with an overwhelming flavor. It is best to avoid sweet wines at the start of a meal, as the sugar content and sweet taste tend to spoil the appetite.

To enhance the taste, serve white wines chilled, but not overly chilled, and red wines at cool room temperature. Open heavy-bodied reds at least an hour before serving, or decant them. Serve either red or white in glasses large enough to let the full bouquet and flavor develop and to let the wine "breathe." When it is poured, first notice the color, then smell the wine. Taste it carefully; roll it against the roof of the mouth to stimulate your taste buds. Then swallow it slowly. Enjoy the difference that a bottle of Italian wine can make to your meal!

WINE IN COOKING

Wine plays a big role in cooking Italian dishes. Even a small amount accentuates the flavor of aromatic herbs and spices and helps to blend all ingredients in a harmonious whole. Wines can add zest to a dish. Often the "secret taste" of some fabulous sauce is the slight accent of wine, which you may be unable to identify in the finished dish.

White wine is used for cooking fish, chicken and veal; it can also be used for poaching eggs and cooking vegetables and risotto. Red wine is great for pasta sauces and for cooking meats, also for poaching fruits and for marinades. Vermouth is used for fish, chicken, salad dressings. Sweet wine, especially Marsala, is used for veal, chicken, beef and desserts. Liqueurs such as Sambuca and Amaretto impart their herbal and botanical flavorings to interesting main-course dishes, and they are used for many desserts.

APPETIZERS,
FIRST COURSES,
SOUPS

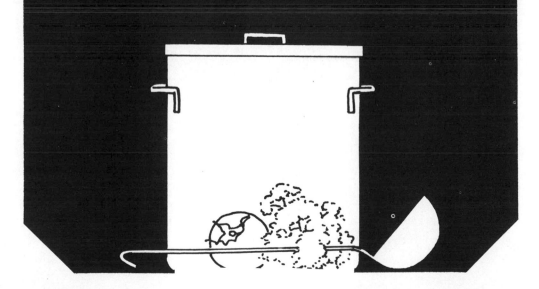

Antipasti are served as the first course in a complete meal in Italy. Translated as "before the pasta," *antipasti* occupy the diner while the chef prepares the pasta. An enormous variety of dishes can be offered, including fruits and vegetables that vary with the seasons and seafood that varies with the region.

On a tray of mixed appetizers one would expect to find these as well as prosciutto (dry-cured Italian ham), cheese and salami. Such *antipasti* make good accompaniments to an *aperitivo*.

The enjoyment of a lunch or dinner should not be hampered by having guests stuffed with heavy cocktail food and hard liquor. Lots of salty snack foods are also a poor choice; they do not stimulate the appetite for the rest of the food, but do exactly the opposite. The usual predinner drinks are also very filling and caloric. Instead, try small amounts of dry wine or an aromatized wine such as vermouth.

The best "appetizers" are raw vegetables with light dips; seafoods with lemon or other light dressings; stuffed small vegetables. This chapter gives only a small selection of these dishes. Most are intended as first courses to be eaten at table; a few can be served as finger food with apéritifs. For additional recipes in other chapters that can be adapted for first-course serving, see the index.

VEGETABLE ANTIPASTO

Vegetables can make an attractive centerpiece as well as a perfect first course. Your guests will delight in such an appetizing beginning, light, tasty, not fattening, and very healthy. Use any of the raw fresh vegetables listed and arrange them in baskets, crystal bowls or oblong serving plates.

> *Mushrooms, sliced thin*
> *Fennel strips*
> *Tomatoes, tiny specimens*
> *Zucchini, thin rounds or slices*
> *Asparagus tips*
> *Broccoli flowerets*
> *Radishes*
> *Cucumber slices or sticks*
> *Carrot sticks*
> *Cauliflowerets*
> *Green beans*

If you have never eaten raw asparagus, broccoli, cauliflower or green beans, this will be a new taste experience for you.

Serve with a choice of dips. Your guests may eat the vegetables plain or with low-calorie dips (following recipes).

CUCUMBER DIP

TIME: 10 MINUTES, EXCLUDING TIME FOR CHILLING
CALORIES: 5 PER TABLESPOON

- 1 *young cucumber, about 8 ounces, or 2 smaller ones, 10 ounces together*
- ¼ *cup liquid skim milk*
- ½ *cup skim-milk cottage or ricotta cheese, or more*
- 2 *tablespoons snipped fresh dill*
- 1 *tablespoon snipped fresh chives*
- 1 *tablespoon prepared Dijon mustard*
  dash of cayenne
  salt

Peel and dice cucumber. Combine all ingredients except salt in a blender container, and blend at low speed for 3 seconds. Switch to high speed for 3 seconds. Taste, and add salt if necessary. Continue to add more cheese until the dip is as thick as you like it. Adjust the amounts of herbs to suit your taste. Chill dip; it will thicken further as it cools. MAKES ABOUT 2 CUPS.

This recipe is a close relative of that for Cold Cucumber Soup, but proportions of liquid to solid are different.

TOMATO-CURRY DIP JOSHI

TIME: 5 MINUTES, EXCLUDING TIME FOR CHILLING
CALORIES: 4 PER TABLESPOON

- 1 *cup fresh Tomato Sauce (p. 245), or 2 medium-size fresh tomatoes, skinned and stewed*
- 1 *tablespoon prepared Dijon mustard*
- 1 *tablespoon curry powder*
- 2 *tablespoons snipped fresh dill*

Put everything in the blender and whirl until smooth. Chill. MAKES 1¼ CUPS.

RICOTTA-EGG DIP DELIAH

TIME: 5 MINUTES, EXCLUDING TIME FOR CHILLING
CALORIES: 13 PER TABLESPOON

½ cup skim-milk ricotta cheese
2 hard-cooked egg yolks
2 tablespoons snipped fresh chives
1 tablespoon prepared Dijon mustard
   pepper

Put everything but pepper in the blender and whirl until smooth. Chill. Add pepper to taste. MAKES ABOUT 1 CUP.

EGGPLANT ALLA JAMAL

TIME: 10 MINUTES, EXCLUDING TIME FOR CHILLING
SERVINGS: 12 OR MORE (3 TABLESPOONS EACH)
CALORIES: 30 PER TABLESPOON

1 eggplant, 1 ½ pounds
2 tablespoons olive oil
1 garlic clove, peeled
6 shallots, peeled
3 tablespoons chopped fresh Italian parsley
2 tablespoons lemon juice
   salt and pepper

Peel eggplant and cut into small cubes. Place them in a single layer on a baking sheet and sprinkle with 1 tablespoon of the oil. Slide under the broiler and broil for 5 minutes. Remove from broiler and let cubes cool. Heat remaining oil in a small skillet and push garlic through a press into the oil. Chop shallots into pan, add parsley, and sauté for 2 minutes. Put eggplant cubes and parsley mixture in a blender container. Add lemon juice, and blend for a few seconds, until the mixture is smooth. Season with salt and pepper to taste. Chill until ready to serve. Serve on Venus crackers, small wheat rounds, or cubes of rye or wheat Italian bread. MAKES ABOUT 2½ CUPS.

VARIATIONS: Instead of bread or crackers as a base, use inch-long sections of celery ribs or whole Belgian endives, or stuff cherry tomatoes with the purée.
   Vary the spread by adding diced green peppers or chopped black olives.

Dice eggplant and steam for 8 minutes. Mash with sautéed ingredients, add lemon juice, and season to taste. This gives a different texture. For creamy texture, add ¼ cup skim-milk ricotta cheese.

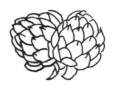

ARTICHOKE CAPONATA ALLA CAVASINO

TIME: 20 MINUTES, EXCLUDING TIME FOR COOKING ARTICHOKES
SERVINGS: 4
CALORIES: 115 PER SERVING

> 2 cooked large fresh artichoke bottoms (p. 195)
> 2 white onions, 1 ounce each
> 2 tablespoons olive oil
> 2 garlic cloves, peeled
> ½ cup dry white wine
> 3 tablespoons capers
> ⅓ teaspoon crumbled dried orégano
>   salt and pepper

When artichoke bottoms are cool enough to handle, remove all remaining leaves and the choke. Cut bottoms into small dice; there should be 1 cup. Peel and mince onions; there should be ¼ cup. Heat oil in a skillet and push garlic through a press into the oil. Add onions and artichoke dice, and sauté for 4 minutes. Add wine, capers and orégano, and cook over low heat, covered, for 10 minutes. Taste, and add salt and pepper if necessary. Serve hot or cold. MAKES ABOUT 2 CUPS.

This makes an excellent appetizer, but it can also serve as a vegetable to accompany a main course, and it can be served as a sauce with risotto or pasta.

SICILIAN CAPONATA BUONAPARTE

TIME: 20 MINUTES
SERVINGS: ABOUT 10 (½ CUP EACH)
CALORIES: 70 PER ½ CUP

 1 *eggplant, about 1 ¼ pounds*
    salt
 2 *large green peppers*
 2 *onions, 4 ounces each*
 ½ *pound fresh plum tomatoes*
 3 *tablespoons olive oil*
 1 *garlic clove, peeled*
 1 *tablespoon red-wine vinegar*
 3 *tablespoons capers*
 ⅓ *teaspoon Italian seasoning*
    pepper
 ⅓ *cup chopped fresh Italian parsley*

Wash and trim eggplant, but do not peel. Cut eggplant into small cubes; there should be about 2 cups. Soak cubes in cold water with 1 tablespoon salt for each quart of water for 10 minutes. Drain, rinse, drain again, and pat dry. While eggplant is soaking, wash and trim peppers, discard ribs and seeds, and chop peppers. Peel and chop onions. Wash tomatoes, discard hard portion near stem, and chop; there should be 1 cup. Heat olive oil in a large skillet and push garlic through a press into the oil. Add onions and sauté until the bits are translucent. Add chopped peppers and dried eggplant cubes, and sauté, stirring often, for 5 minutes. Add vinegar, capers and Italian seasoning, and cook for 2 or 3 minutes. Add tomatoes and cook for 5 minutes longer. Taste, and add salt and pepper if needed. Stir in the parsley. Serve warm or cold. MAKES 5 TO 6 CUPS.

ASPARAGUS-STUFFED EGGS

TIME: 10 MINUTES
SERVINGS: 4 (2 HALVES PER SERVING)
CALORIES: 90 PER SERVING

 6 *fresh asparagus*
 4 *hard-cooked eggs*
 ¼ *cup fresh lemon juice*
 1 *teaspoon minced fresh tarragon*
 1 *garlic clove, peeled and crushed*
    salt and pepper
 1 *pimiento, cut into strips*

Wash and trim asparagus, and break off the tough portion of the stalks. Blanch or steam asparagus for 5 to 6 minutes, and drain well. Shell eggs and cut lengthwise into halves. Put the yolk portion into a blender container with the asparagus, lemon juice, tarragon and garlic. Blend for a few seconds, until reduced to a purée. Season the purée with salt and pepper to taste. Stuff the egg whites, and garnish with pimiento strips.

MOZZARELLA AND TOMATO SALAD

TIME: 5 MINUTES
SERVINGS: 6
CALORIES: 80 PER SERVING

    4 large firm ripe tomatoes, 1 ½ pounds altogether
    1 pound skim-milk mozzarella cheese
    1 tablespoon vegetable oil
    2 tablespoons chopped fresh basil
    2 tablespoons chopped fresh Italian parsley
       salt and freshly ground pepper

Wash tomatoes and cut into thin round slices. Cut mozzarella into slices of the same shape. Sprinkle oil over the tomato slices, and arrange cheese and tomato slices on 6 plates. Sprinkle basil and parsley over cheese and tomato slices, and salt and pepper to taste.

GNOCCHI ALLA CELLI

TIME: 20 MINUTES
SERVINGS: 9
CALORIES: 110 PER SERVING

Make Strozzapreti (p. 48). When spinach drops have been poached, lift to a plate and let them cool a little. Then turn into a bowl and toss with small amounts of melted butter and grated Parmesan cheese. Use 4 or 5 for a first-course serving.

VARIATIONS: Plain tomato sauce or cheese sauce can be used instead of butter and Parmesan.

ANCHOVY MUSHROOMS FRANCESCO

TIME: 10 MINUTES
SERVINGS: 8 (3 MUSHROOMS EACH)
CALORIES: 20 PER MUSHROOM

24 *large fresh mushrooms*
 6 *flat anchovy fillets*
¾ *cup skim-milk ricotta cheese*
    juice of 1 lemon
 3 *tablespoons minced fresh Italian parsley*
    black pepper
¼ *cup grated Parmesan cheese*

Wash and trim mushrooms. Remove stems and set caps aside; mince the stems. Mince and mash anchovies until they are almost puréed. Stir them into the ricotta cheese and add minced mushroom stems, lemon juice and parsley. Season with black pepper to taste. Carefully fill mushroom caps, rounding the filling slightly in the center. Sprinkle ½ teaspoon Parmesan cheese over each mushroom. Slide under a preheated broiler and broil for 5 minutes, until mushrooms are hot and cheese golden. Serve hot, 3 mushrooms per serving, or arrange as part of a tray of *antipasti*.

CRAB-FILLED MUSHROOMS

TIME: 20 MINUTES
SERVINGS: 8 (3 MUSHROOMS EACH)
CALORIES: 28 PER MUSHROOM

24 *large fresh mushrooms*
1½ *tablespoons unsalted butter*
 1 *cup fresh crab meat*
    juice of 1 lemon
 3 *tablespoons dry Marsala wine*
¼ *cup chopped fresh Italian parsley*
    salt and pepper
½ *cup shredded skim-milk mozzarella cheese*
    oil for baking dish

Wash and trim mushrooms. Remove stems and set caps aside. Chop the stems and sauté in the butter, covered, over medium heat for 3 minutes. Pick over the crab meat carefully to remove any bits of cartilage, and mix crab with lemon juice, wine, parsley and sautéed mushroom stems. Add salt and pepper to taste. Carefully fill mushroom caps, rounding the filling slightly in the center. Divide mozzarella among the mushrooms so each little cap has an even layer of cheese, about 1 teaspoon per mushroom. Arrange in an oiled baking dish and cover the dish, but try not to touch the tops of the mushrooms. Bake in a preheated 400°F. oven for 8 minutes; the mushrooms should be very hot, the cheese melted and golden. Serve hot, 3 mushrooms per serving, plain, or on a bed of minced parsley. Or arrange as part of a tray of *antipasti*.

VARIATION: Sprinkle tops with grated Parmesan cheese.

ZUCCHINI CUPS FILLED WITH MUSHROOMS ALLA ALITALIA

TIME: 15 MINUTES
SERVINGS: 24 CUPS
CALORIES: 25 PER CUP

    4 *fat zucchini, each about 7 inches long*
      salt
    4 *ounces fresh mushrooms*
    4 *ounces red pimientos, drained*
    1 *tablespoon vegetable oil*
    ¼ *cup chopped fresh Italian parsley*
      pepper
    3 *hard-cooked eggs, or 8 pitted olives, or 24 pimiento strips, or a*
      mixture

Scrub zucchini, but do not peel; cut off ends, and cut zucchini into 1-inch-long sections, about 6 from each zucchini. Cover with cold water and add 1 teaspoon salt; bring to a boil, and simmer for 2 or 3 minutes; the pieces should still be crisp. Hollow out the centers of the pieces, keeping the bottom of each piece unbroken. Chop the scooped-out pulp and set aside. Wash and trim mushrooms, and chop to fine pieces. Chop pimientos. Heat the oil in a skillet and sauté the pulp, mushrooms, pimientos and parsley for a few minutes, only until everything is tender and well mixed, but not mushy. Season with salt and pepper to taste. Put about 1 tablespoon of the filling into each zucchini cup. Slice the eggs or olives. Garnish each cup with an egg slice or an olive slice or a pimiento strip, or use some of each to have variety. Serve for party food, or have several pieces for a first-course serving.

ZUCCHINI PANCAKES

TIME: 10 TO 15 MINUTES, EXCLUDING TIME TO REST THE BATTER
SERVINGS: ABOUT 16 PANCAKES
CALORIES: 40 PER PANCAKE

> 4 *small zucchini, about 4 ounces each*
> 3 *eggs*
> ¼ *cup water*
> ¼ *cup whole-wheat flour*
> 3 *tablespoons chopped fresh Italian parsley*
> *salt and pepper*
> 2 *tablespoons vegetable oil*

Wash and peel zucchini, cut into chunks, and purée in the blender. Beat eggs lightly in a bowl and add zucchini, water, flour, parsley, and a tiny pinch of salt and pepper. Return the mixture to the blender and whirl for a few seconds, until well mixed; batter does not need to be as smooth as cream. For best results let the batter rest in a cool place for 1 hour, but this is not essential.

Brush a 5-inch skillet with a few drops of the oil, and heat the pan until a drop of water skips across the pan. Spoon 3 tablespoons of the batter into the skillet and quickly turn and tip the pan so the batter fills the entire surface. Cook until the top shows little holes and the bottom is lightly browned, a few minutes. Flip over and brown the other side. Remove to a plate and keep warm. Continue to brush the pan with a few drops of the oil and make pancakes until all the batter is used.

VARIATIONS: To make less of a pancake and more of a *frittata,*, omit whole-wheat flour and add 3 more eggs (which will increase calories). Serve the little *frittatas* plain or filled.

Fill pancakes or *frittatas* with seafood, vegetable mixtures, meat sauce, rice and chicken, mushrooms and mozzarella cheese, and roll up like a crêpe; or make layers as if making a layer cake, and serve cut into wedges.

Top either pancakes or *frittatas* with tomato sauce and cheese.

TOMATOES STUFFED WITH SHRIMPS BARBARA

TIME: 20 MINUTES
SERVINGS: 4 (2 TOMATOES PER SERVING)
CALORIES: 60 PER 1 TOMATO

8 medium-size tomatoes, 1 ½ pounds altogether
½ pound small shrimps in shells
1 tablespoon vegetable oil
3 shallots, peeled
3 tablespoons chopped fresh Italian parsley
3 tablespoons lemon juice
5 tablespoons snipped fresh dill
½ cup skim-milk ricotta cheese
   salt and pepper

Wash tomatoes, and cut a small slice off the top of each. Carefully scoop out the pulp and let it drain in a strainer. Turn the tomato shells upside down to drain. Shell and devein the shrimps and poach them for 5 minutes, until they are pink; do not overcook. Heat the oil in a skillet and chop the shallots into the pan. Add parsley and sauté until shallots are translucent. Add drained tomato pulp, shrimps, lemon juice and dill, and cook for 3 minutes. Add ricotta and cook for 5 minutes longer. Season with salt and pepper to taste. Divide the filling among the tomato shells. Place them under the broiler for 5 minutes, then serve at once.

SHRIMPS MARSALA ALLA ENNIO

TIME: 15 MINUTES
SERVINGS: 4
CALORIES: 150 PER SERVING

16 medium-size raw shrimps in shells
 2 tablespoons unsalted butter
 3 shallots, peeled
½ garlic clove, peeled (optional)
 3 tablespoons dry white wine
½ cup dry Marsala wine
    juice of 1 lemon
½ teaspoon Italian seasoning
    salt and black pepper
¼ cup chopped fresh Italian parsley

Peel shrimps and devein if necessary. Melt butter in a medium-size saucepan. Chop shallots into the pan and put garlic (if you use it) through a press into pan. Add shrimps and sauté for 5 minutes. Add white wine, Marsala, lemon juice and Italian seasoning. Cook for 5 minutes longer. Season with salt and pepper to taste. Serve in shallow bowls, sprinkled with parsley.

VARIATION: Instead of butter, white wine and Marsala, use vegetable oil and ¼ cup red wine with ½ cup tomato sauce.

FISH ALLA TERESA

Use striped bass, bluefish or flounder. Poach the fish in water with herbs for 6 minutes, or until tender (the size and thickness of the fish will determine the exact number of minutes). Cool, then remove all skin and bones and flake the fish. For each pound of flaked fish prepare ¼ cup Salsa alla Teresa (p. 254). Arrange fish on a serving platter, spoon the sauce over, and garnish with parsley sprigs and lemon slices. Or arrange individual amounts of the fish and spoon 1 tablespoon of the sauce over each serving.

EGGPLANT STUFFED WITH SHRIMPS AND MUSHROOMS

TIME: 20 MINUTES
SERVINGS: 4 AS MAIN DISH, 8 AS FIRST COURSE
CALORIES: 240 PER MAIN-COURSE SERVING, 120 PER FIRST-COURSE
            SERVING

2 *eggplants, 1 pound each*
1 *pound fresh mushrooms*
1 *pound raw shrimps in shells*
2 *tablespoons vegetable oil*
1 *onion, 4 ounces, peeled*
2 *garlic cloves, peeled*
¼ *cup chopped fresh Italian parsley*
½ *cup dry white wine*
¼ *teaspoon Italian seasoning*
   salt and pepper
3 *tablespoons grated Parmesan cheese*

Wash eggplants and remove stems and leaves, but do not peel. Cut lengthwise into halves, and carefully scoop out the pulp without damaging the shells. Poach the shells in a large pot of water for 5 minutes, then turn upside down to drain. Wash and trim the mushrooms, dry in paper towels, then chop into coarse pieces. Shell and devein the raw shrimps, and chop them. Oil a large baking dish with a few drops of the oil, and heat the rest in a large skillet. Chop onion into the oil and push the garlic through a press into the pan. Add mushrooms and the scooped-out eggplant pulp. When onion is translucent and the other vegetables just tender, a few minutes, add chopped shrimps, 2 tablespoons of the parsley, the wine and Italian seasoning. Cook for 5 minutes, stirring often to mix. Taste and add salt and pepper. Place eggplant shells in the oiled baking dish and fill them with the shrimp mixture. Sprinkle the tops with the rest of the parsley and the cheese. Place under the broiler for a few minutes longer, until cheese is golden brown. Serve 1 eggplant half for a main dish. Cut each half again into halves for a first-course serving.

VARIATION: Instead of mushrooms and white wine, use 1 pound fresh plum tomatoes. Wash them, cut out hard portion near stem, and chop into small pieces. Add to chopped eggplant pulp and cook until just tender.

Other filling possibilities are diced cooked meat or chicken, or mixed vegetables.

STRIPED BASS WITH VERMOUTH DRESSING

TIME: 15 MINUTES
SERVINGS: 8
CALORIES: 145 PER SERVING

2 fillets of striped bass, 1 pound each
1 tablespoon vegetable oil
2 lemons
1 tablespoon prepared Dijon mustard
3 tablespoons dry white vermouth
    salt and pepper
2 shallots, peeled
4 sprigs of Italian parsley
8 lettuce leaves

Rinse fillets and pat dry. Cut each fillet into 4 pieces. Put pieces in a shallow pan; add the oil and enough water to cover. Bring to a boil and poach over medium heat for 8 minutes. Remove pan from heat, drain, and cool. While fish is poaching, mix in a small bowl the juice of 1 lemon, the mustard, vermouth, and salt and pepper to taste. Cut the shallots into rings and chop the parsley. Arrange 1 lettuce leaf on each of 8 plates. Arrange 1 piece of fish on each lettuce leaf. Spoon even amounts of dressing over the fish and garnish with the shallot rings, parsley, and the remaining lemon cut into thin wedges. Serve warm or cold.

FISH SALAD PESCARA

TIME: 15 MINUTES, EXCLUDING TIME FOR CHILLING
SERVINGS: 6
CALORIES: 160 PER SERVING (BASED ON STRIPED BASS)

    1 ½ pounds filleted fresh saltwater fish
    ½ pound fresh plum tomatoes
    ½ cup chopped shallots
    ¼ cup chopped fresh Italian parsley
    2 garlic cloves, peeled
    1 tablespoon olive oil
    ¼ cup fresh lemon juice
    2 tablespoons drained capers
    2 bay leaves
       salt and pepper

Cut fish into 1-inch cubes and poach in a small amount of water for 6 minutes. Drain and cool. Wash tomatoes, remove hard portion near stem, and chop; there should be 1 cup. Pour tomatoes into a large mixing bowl and add shallots and parsley. Push garlic through a press into the bowl. Add fish cubes and olive oil, and toss gently to mix. Add lemon juice, capers, bay leaves, and salt and pepper to taste. Chill. Remove bay leaves before serving.

VARIATION: Heat oil in a skillet, push garlic through a press into oil, and add shallots and chopped tomatoes. Cook for 5 minutes. Add parsley, lemon juice, capers, bay leaves and fish cubes. Cook for 5 minutes longer, until fish is just tender. Season to taste, remove bay leaves, and serve warm.

COLD SEAFOOD RUGGERO

TIME: 15 MINUTES, EXCLUDING TIME FOR CHILLING
SERVINGS: 6
CALORIES: 115 PER SERVING

> 6 fresh mussels in shells
> 12 raw shrimps in shells
> ½ cup diced fresh raw squid
> ½ cup cooked fresh crab meat
> 3 pimientos, drained
> 6 shallots, peeled
> ⅓ cup chopped fresh Italian parsley
> ¼ cup chopped celery
> 1 garlic clove, peeled
> 2 tablespoons vegetable oil
> 2 tablespoons red-wine vinegar
> juice of 2 lemons
> ¼ teaspoon Italian seasoning
> salt and freshly ground black pepper

Scrub mussels, remove beards, and steam over a small amount of water until shells open, about 4 minutes. Remove mussels from shells and place in a bowl. Poach shrimps in enough water to cover until shells turn pink, about 5 minutes. Remove shells, devein if necessary, and chop shrimps into ½-inch pieces. Add to the mussels. Poach the squid pieces in water to cover for 2 or 3 minutes; do not overcook the squid or it will toughen. Drain squid and add to the mussels and shrimps. (All the steaming and poaching steps can be done at the same time.) Add the crab meat. Let all the seafood cool.

Chop the pimientos and shallots into a large salad bowl. Add parsley and celery, and push the garlic through a press into the vegetables. Add cooled seafood and the oil, and toss to mix. Then pour in vinegar and lemon juice and add Italian seasoning and salt and pepper to taste. Toss again to mix well, and serve well chilled.

For large groups the ingredients can be increased to make more servings; it is an excellent dish for a buffet. Although this is a perfect first course, it can serve as a main dish or as a salad.

CHICKEN LIVER CROSTINI DINI

TIME: 12 MINUTES
SERVINGS: 8 TO 10
CALORIES: 20 PER TABLESPOON

½ *pound chicken livers*
  salt
2 *hard-cooked eggs*
1 *tablespoon prepared Dijon mustard*
3 *tablespoons skim-milk ricotta cheese*
1 *tablespoon Marsala wine*
2 *tablespoons snipped fresh chives*
2 *small shallots, peeled and chopped*
  black pepper

Simmer chicken livers in 1 cup water with ½ teaspoon salt for 8 minutes. Drain. While livers are cooking, shell eggs and mash. Put livers and mashed eggs into a blender container and add mustard, cheese, wine, chives, shallots, and black pepper to taste. Blend at high speed for 1 second, then at low speed for 1 second. If the mixture is not as smooth as you like, whirl again for 1 second.

With a spatula push the pâté into a bowl or crock. Serve with celery strips or wheat crackers or whole-wheat bread, cut into squares and toasted in the broiler.

CROSTINI PROVATURA ALLA RUSSO

TIME: 15 MINUTES
SERVINGS: 8 SQUARES
CALORIES: 50 PER SQUARE

2 *pieces of bread, toasted*
2 *slices of medium-size fresh mozzarella cheese, made from*
   buffalo's milk, or 3 slices of whole-milk cow's-milk mozzarella
1 *tablespoon unsalted butter*
2 *anchovy fillets*
3 *tablespoons minced fresh Italian parsley*

Cut the pieces of toast into 4 squares each, and arrange them in a single layer in a baking dish. (Baking dish can be coated with nonstick lining or rubbed with a few drops of oil.) Cut mozzarella to fit the toast squares. Melt butter in a small saucepan over low heat. Snip anchovies into butter, making very small bits. Add parsley and heat until anchovies are melted; mash them with a wooden spoon to help the process. Pour sauce over the bread slices. Bake the *crostini* in a preheated 350°F. oven for 5 minutes, or slide under the broiler for a few minutes.

SOUPS

MINESTRE E ZUPPE

Italian soup, *minestra* or *zuppa*, can be a light first course in a meal or a hearty main course.

Main-course soups include *minestrone*, a thick vegetable soup, usually with rice or pasta in it, and *zuppa di pesche*, made with various fishes and shellfishes. (For main-course fish soups see the index.) Also there are main-course soups made with beans and pasta in a tomato-sauce base, soups based on meat or chicken, and beef with vegetables, a favorite on a cold day.

Clear soups, *minestrini*, are made of either beef or chicken stock. When various forms of pasta or *pastina*, very small shapes of pasta, are added, it becomes *pasta in brodo*. When clear consommés are simmered to make them stronger and more concentrated, they are referred to as *ristretti* (reduced), or *doppio* (double strength). If beaten eggs are stirred into the soup, it is called *stracciatella* (in rags). If a whole poached egg on a piece of fried bread is added, it is *pavese*.

Many soups based on puréed vegetables, such as *crema di asparagi* or *crema di funghi* (mushroom), are popular as first courses.

All the right seasonings and finishing touches are important. Fresh herbs make a big difference in the flavor of a good soup. Don't forget the final touch—the topping of grated Parmesan cheese. Use small soup bowls, and warm them before pouring in the soup. If the soup is just the beginning for the meal, serve small portions; the soup is not designed to satisfy the appetite but to start the processes of digestion so that the meal that follows is enjoyed to the full. Coordinate the soup with the rest of the meal so that it complements and enhances the main course.

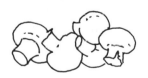

STOCK

Homemade stock takes time to prepare, but when completed it can be stored in refrigerator or freezer, ready for use in soups and sauces. Your own stock can be as flavorful as you like, and as lightly salted as you like, an advantage over most commercial stocks. Meat stocks need long cooking, but a useful vegetable stock can be ready in 30 minutes.

CHICKEN STOCK, ITALIAN STYLE

TIME: 2 HOURS
CALORIES: 30 PER CUP

    4 pounds chicken parts (bones, necks, backs, wings)
    3 leeks
    3 celery ribs
    1 ripe red tomato, 5 ounces
    1 carrot
    1 white onion, 1 ounce
    2 teaspoons peppercorns, crushed
    5 sprigs of Italian parsley
    1 teaspoon fresh or dried thyme
    1 bay leaf
    ¼ teaspoon Italian seasoning

Rinse chicken parts well and put them into a large stockpot. Wash, scrape, or peel the vegetables, and chop into the stockpot. Add peppercorns, herbs and Italian seasoning. Pour in enough water to reach 1 inch above the ingredients. Cover the pot and bring to a boil. Reduce heat, and simmer for about 2 hours. With a fork remove the chicken pieces and put aside. Strain everything else in the stockpot through a sieve lined with dampened cheese-cloth into a bowl. Chill the strained stock.

    When the stock is cold, lift off the fat that has risen to the surface. Transfer the stock to jars for refrigerator storage, or pour into 1-cup containers or into an ice-cube tray for freezer storage. When completely frozen, the cubes can be transferred to a plastic freezer bag; use the cubes a few at a time, as you need them. MAKES ABOUT 2 QUARTS.

    The chicken meat can be used for any dish requiring poached chicken. Discard bones, skin, tendons, etc. Serve sprinkled with lemon juice, or sauced with Salsa Verde (p. 243).

    My mother's secret for superior chicken stock: add a small chunk of Parmesan or pecorino cheese (about 1½ ounces) to the chicken stock for flavoring.

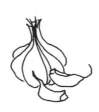

VEAL STOCK

TIME: 6 HOURS
CALORIES: 35 PER CUP

3 pounds meaty veal bones (shanks, knuckles)
1 onion, 4 ounces
2 whole cloves
1 large carrot
½ cup chopped Italian parsley stems
1 bay leaf
2 coriander berries, crushed
½ pound boneless veal from breast, shoulder or flank
½ teaspoon Italian seasoning
2 teaspoons salt

Put veal bones in a large stockpot (8 quarts is the ideal size). Cover with cold water, bring to a boil, and boil for 5 minutes, skimming often. Pour off the water; rinse veal pieces and the pot. Return the bones to the pot and pour in 4 quarts cold water. Peel onion, stick cloves into it, and add to the stockpot. Wash and scrape carrot and cut into chunks; add to stockpot with parsley stems, bay leaf and coriander berries. Again bring to a boil. Then reduce to a simmer, half-cover the pot, and cook for 5 to 6 hours. During the first hour skim the stock often. After 4 hours, add the boneless veal, Italian seasoning and salt. Taste stock after 5 hours; it should be flavorful; if not, cook for the extra hour. Let stock rest for 10 minutes, then ladle it through a coarse strainer. All vegetables and herbs will be flavorless, so discard them. The boneless veal and any scraps of meat from the bones can be saved for stuffing vegetables. Pour the stock through a fine strainer lined with dampened cheesecloth, and chill it. Discard any fat that has risen to the top. Stock will keep in the refrigerator for at least 5 days, or it can be frozen in 1-cup jars or freezer trays. MAKES ABOUT 2 QUARTS.

VEGETABLE STOCK

TIME: 30 MINUTES
CALORIES: 10 PER CUP

4 cups water
1 cup chopped vegetables
2 tablespoons chopped fresh Italian parsley
½ teaspoon minced fresh basil
¼ teaspoon Italian seasoning
   salt and pepper

VEGETABLES: Use 2 or 3 kinds of vegetables, according to the season. Choose from carrots, celery, leeks, onions, potatoes, tomatoes, zucchini. Wash, peel if necessary, and cut into small bits.

Pour water into a large saucepan and add vegetables, herbs and Italian seasoning. Cover and simmer for about 30 minutes. Season with salt and pepper to taste. Use as is, for a simple soup, or purée, or strain and clarify. MAKES ABOUT 4 CUPS CLEAR SOUP.

CLARIFYING STOCK

Pour 5 cups defatted strained stock into a 2-quart pot. Separate 2 eggs. Use the yolks for another recipe. Crumble shells and drop into stock. Beat egg whites lightly, just until well mixed, and pour into stock. Bring stock very slowly to a simmer, stirring with a wooden spoon or paddle, and let the pot barely simmer for about 45 minutes. Don't stop stirring. If it is difficult to keep the temperature low enough, set the pot over an asbestos mat. With a skimmer lift off most of the egg mass on top, then ladle the stock through a fine sieve lined with dampened cheesecloth. MAKES ABOUT 4 CUPS CLARI-FIED STOCK.

STROZZAPRETI
(spinach soup drops)

For a delicate garnish to any clear soup use 2 or 3 spinach drops. Add to clear chicken stock or to vegetable stock. To use for a first course, see page 35.

TIME: 15 TO 20 MINUTES
SERVINGS: 9 (5 DROPS PER SERVING)
CALORIES: 17 PER DROP

1 ½ pounds fresh spinach
3 eggs
½ cup grated Parmesan cheese
⅓ cup fresh crumbs from whole-wheat Italian bread

Wash spinach thoroughly, remove stems and any damaged leaves, and cook in the water clinging to the leaves for 5 minutes. Drain thoroughly, then chop very fine; there should be 2 cups. Beat eggs in a bowl and add spinach, half of the cheese, and enough of the crumbs to make a stiff paste. Using about 1 tablespoon at a time, make tiny balls, like meatballs, of the mixture. Roll them in the rest of the cheese, spread on a sheet of wax paper. Fill a large pot with water, bring to a boil, and drop in the spinach balls. Simmer for only a few minutes, then lift out with a skimmer.

ESCAROLE SOUP WITH EGG THREADS

TIME: 15 TO 20 MINUTES
SERVINGS: 4
CALORIES: 105 PER SERVING

1 pound fresh escarole
3 cups chicken stock
½ teaspoon Italian seasoning
¼ cup grated Parmesan cheese
2 large eggs, slightly beaten

Wash the escarole in several changes of water and remove root ends and any damaged leaves. Steam over 1 cup water until tender, about 5 minutes. Chop to very small pieces and turn into a large saucepan with the chicken stock, Italian seasoning and cheese. Bring to a simmer, stirring. Still stirring, pour in the eggs; they should form into threads as you stir and begin to cook at once. As soon as the egg threads are cooked to your taste, remove from heat and serve, with extra cheese on the side.

TOMATO, SPINACH, MUSHROOM SOUP

TIME: 15 TO 20 MINUTES
SERVINGS: 4 (SCANT 1 CUP EACH)
CALORIES: 85 PER SERVING

1 pound fresh plum tomatoes
¾ pound fresh spinach
¼ pound fresh mushrooms
1 garlic clove, peeled
½ teaspoon grated nutmeg
¼ cup grated Parmesan cheese
1 cup water
salt and pepper

Wash and peel tomatoes and chop; there should be 2 cups. Wash spinach thoroughly, remove stems and any damaged leaves, and cook in the water clinging to the leaves for 4 minutes. Drain and chop spinach; there should be 1 cup. Wash and trim mushrooms and chop; there should be ½ cup. Put all vegetables in a saucepan, and push garlic through a press into the mixture. Add nutmeg, cheese and water. Cover the pan and simmer over medium-low heat for 10 minutes. Add salt and pepper to taste.

TOMATO AND ZUCCHINI SOUP

TIME: 20 MINUTES
SERVINGS: 6 (SCANT 1 CUP EACH)
CALORIES: 40 PER SERVING WITHOUT CHEESE

    1 pound fresh plum tomatoes
    3 shallots, peeled
    4 zucchini, 5 ounces each
    ⅓ cup chopped fresh Italian parsley
    ⅓ teaspoon Italian seasoning
    1 cup water
       salt and pepper
    6 tablespoons grated Parmesan cheese (optional)

Wash and peel tomatoes, cut into 6 pieces each, and drop into a blender container. Chop shallots into the tomatoes, and whirl the blender for a few seconds to make a purée. Scrub and trim zucchini but do not peel; chop into small bits. Put vegetables, parsley, Italian seasoning and water in a saucepan. Cover and cook over medium heat for 10 minutes, or until zucchini is as tender as you like it. Add salt and pepper to taste. Serve with 1 tablespoon cheese for each serving if you like.

VARIATION: For a perfectly smooth texture, the zucchini can also be puréed in the blender.

COLD CUCUMBER SOUP

TIME: 6 MINUTES, EXCLUDING TIME FOR CHILLING
SERVINGS: 4
CALORIES: 55 PER SERVING

1 *medium-size cucumber*
1 *cup liquid skim milk*
½ *cup skim-milk cottage or ricotta cheese*
2 *tablespoons lemon juice*
¼ *cup snipped fresh dill*
2 *tablespoons snipped fresh chives*
1 *sprig of Italian parsley, snipped*
½ *tablespoon prepared Dijon mustard*
  salt

Peel and dice the cucumber. Combine all ingredients except salt in a blender container, and blend at low speed for 3 seconds. Switch to high speed for 3 seconds. Taste, and add salt or more dill. Chill.

VARIATIONS: To dress up this famous cold summer soup, add a small dab of sour cream on top, and sprinkle with more snipped chives and dill.
  Serve as a delicious sauce for fish or veal.

TRACI'S GAZPACHO

TIME: 20 MINUTES, EXCLUDING TIME FOR CHILLING
SERVINGS: 6
CALORIES: 105 PER SERVING

3 *large tomatoes*
1 *medium-size cucumber*
1 *medium-size onion*
1 *large green pepper*
1 *garlic clove*
2 *eggs*
¾ *cup tomato juice*
3 *tablespoons white-wine vinegar*
2 *tablespoons olive oil*
  juice of 1 lemon
½ *teaspoon prepared Dijon mustard*
¼ *teaspoon cayenne pepper*
  salt
6 *tablespoons watercress leaves*
6 *lemon wedges*

Wash and peel tomatoes, and remove hard portion near the stem. Wash and trim cucumber. Peel the onion. Wash and trim green pepper and discard ribs

Pasta is one of the most popular foods in the world. The hundreds of varieties, the enormous number of sauces, the nutritional value, the ease of preparation—pasta is truly versatile. No proper Italian meal can begin without its *primo piatto,* or first dish: pasta.

It is tiresome to be obliged to defend pasta against the charge that it is fattening. (Actually, the remark "I don't eat pasta often, it's so fattening," heard so often, gave a major impulse toward writing this book.) Pasta can be fattening as it is made, cooked and served in America, but that is American-Italian pasta, not Italian. In Italy pasta is only one course in a meal; it is served by itself and only in small amounts. After pasta come fish or meat, vegetables, salad and fruit.

"Pasta" is the general term for a multitude of forms of dough made of semolina, the refined inner kernels of hard, durum wheat, ground into a semifine flour. The flour is mixed with water and made into a stiff dough which is turned out in hundreds of different machine-made shapes and then dried; this dough makes spaghetti, macaroni, rigatoni, vermicelli. When the flour is mixed with water and eggs and made into a soft dough that is tender and somewhat moist, it will be cut into flat ribbon shapes of varying widths —fettuccine, linguine, tagliarini. The flat ribbons are more familiar to us as "noodles." Pasta can be white, light brown when made with whole wheat, yellow when made with egg (egg noodles), or green when made with spinach.

Pasta is divided into two main categories: *pasta* or *pastina in brodo,* that is pasta cooked and served in broth; and *pasta asciutta,* dry pasta, which includes spaghetti, macaroni, noodles, ravioli, served in sauces.

Pastina comes in dozens of different tiny patterns—circles, squares, shells, stars; all of these are cooked and served in soups.

Dry pasta is made in several basic shapes and in many sizes of these shapes.

1. FLAT RIBBON NOODLES: *fettuccine, lasagne, linguine, tagliarini, tagliatelle,* etc.
2. SOLID LONG RODS: *spaghetti, tonnarelli, vermicelli, capellini,* etc.
3. HOLLOW RODS OR CYLINDERS: *bucatini, maccheroni* (what we call macaroni), *penne, rigatoni,* etc., which may be long or short forms.
4. STUFFED SHAPES: *agnolotti, ravioli, tortellini,* which are formed into small pockets, then stuffed and sealed; or *cannelloni* or *manicotti,* which are sheets stuffed and rolled or large tubes.
5. VARIOUS OTHER SHAPES: *conchiglie* (shells), *farfalle* (butterflies), *fusilli* (spirals), *orecchiette* (ear-shaped), etc.

It is not true that Marco Polo brought pasta to Italy from his travels to China. Pasta was eaten in the peninsula long before that. The Romans served a form of fettuccine with cheese called *laganum cum caseo*. There are statues, tributes, awards for the best pasta creations, even several museums; many pasta factories have exhibitions, and there is a special Museo Storica degli Spaghetti in Pontedassio near the Italian Riviera. Italians scarcely hold their art and music higher than their national dish.

Good pasta cooks and tastes better than inferior brands. Because of the abundance of durum wheat produced in the United States, it is becoming one of the leading producers of pasta. Naturally, the best pasta is still made in Italy. Many authorities believe the best is made in Fara San Martino in Abruzzi.

A serving of 2 ounces of most kinds of pasta (weighed in its dry, uncooked state) produces 210 calories. (There are some whole-wheat pastas that produce fewer calories, but they are not yet available generally.) Pasta, a low-fat food (1.5 percent) and a valuable source of protein (15 percent), contains eight of the essential amino acids. (The pasta sauce generally provides the other amino acids that are necessary for human growth and maintenance.) Pasta also contains B vitamins (thiamin, riboflavin, niacin) and minerals (calcium and iron). It is superior to potatoes in energy-giving carbohydrates. Dr. Ancel Keys, consultant to the World Health Organization (WHO) and the Food and Agriculture Organization (FAO) of the United Nations, has noted in two books that the Italians, on a diet of pasta, have lower serum cholesterol values than Americans and also a very low death rate from heart attacks.

If your idea of pasta is only spaghetti with meatballs, macaroni and cheese, and fettuccine Alfredo, read this chapter. If you can think only of thick red sauce, heavy with meat and oil, read this chapter. In addition to those hundreds of shapes and sizes of pasta, there are hundreds of sauces. Many of them have no meat and little fat or oil. You can create your own style of service and your own versions of the sauces, or invent brand-new ones. Actually, you could serve pasta every day of the year without duplicating a sauce. Even though pasta is the *primo piatto* in Italy, you can serve it as a main course, with salad, cheese and fruit, and a good Italian wine to accompany the meal. A totally satisfying meal, quick to prepare, nutritionally adequate.

HOW TO COOK PASTA

Pasta is a perfect food for the cook with limited time. Most types will be fully cooked in less than 10 minutes, and there are many sauces that can be prepared in less than 15 minutes. The thicker or larger the pasta, the longer it will require, but even thick kinds will be cooked just right in less time than you may have thought.

One pound of pasta will make 8 ample servings. If used as a first course, the portions should be smaller.

Before you start to boil water for the pasta, have everything else ready —the ingredients for the sauce you plan to make, the warmed serving bowl, the grated cheese, and so on. Pasta, like a soufflé, should be served when ready. Therefore, start making the sauce as soon as you start to boil water for pasta. Or start even sooner with the sauce if your pasta is a thin kind that cooks in 4 minutes or less.

Have ready a very large pot with a cover. For 1 pound of pasta use an 8-quart pot. Pour in 6 quarts of water, cover the pot, and bring the water to a rapid boil. Uncover the pot, add 1 tablespoon salt (or omit salt entirely if you prefer), stir, and add the pasta, little by little, so that the boiling does not stop. With a large fork stir all the strands in the pot and let them cook, uncovered, for 6 to 8 minutes for regular spaghetti. The ideal state to achieve is *al dente*, to the tooth; that is, the strand of pasta should be chewable, not mushy. After 6 minutes pull a strand from the pot and chew it to test. Stop cooking at once if it's just right, or cook for a minute or two longer if needed. Do not overcook or the pasta will become too soft.

Immediately remove the pot from the heat and pour the pasta into a large colander or strainer set in the sink. Don't stand directly over the colander as you pour, for steam will rise from the hot contents. Don't rinse the pasta, just let the excess water drain off. Return pasta to the cooking pot, or preferably place in a warmed large serving dish or bowl.

A second way to combine pasta and sauce is the *al segreto* method. Cook pasta for 2 minutes less than *al dente*, drain but do not rinse, toss with butter and cheese, then add to some of the sauce simmering in a large skillet. Cook over low heat, stirring to mix well, for 2 to 3 minutes. Add more cheese and sauce before serving. This method gives pasta more flavor of the sauce. Also, it can be made in advance, then cooked for 2 or 3 minutes just before serving.

The best pasta bowl is a specially made large shallow bowl with a projecting flat edge to make it easy to mix the pasta. Heat the bowl in a low oven, or place briefly on top of the boiling pasta pot to warm. Pasta must be kept warm: once cooled, the gluten in the flour makes the strands stick together and become gummy. To prevent this, in addition to serving it hot, have butter or oil in the bottom of the warmed dish; this will keep the pasta from sticking to the dish or to itself. At once turn the strands over to coat them with butter or oil. If you like, you may also have in the dish some grated cheese and a few spoons of sauce. With two forks toss together quickly.

Now add the sauce or grated cheese, little by little, and continue to toss with the forks until you reach the consistency you prefer. The balance of the sauce and cheese will be served separately at table for each person to add as he chooses.

If you are cooking a few tablespoons of pastina, you won't need an

8-quart pot, but if you plan to prepare 2 or 3 pounds of pasta, you'll need a proportionately larger kettle, or several pots. Adjust the size of the pot, amount of water and salt to the amount of pasta you are cooking, but always use a large enough pot so that your pasta will be whirled around in ample water that is boiling rapidly.

Pastas other than regular spaghetti will require slightly different times. Thin spaghetti or spaghettini, vermicelli, thin linguine or capellini will be cooked in less time, 4 to 5 minutes; thicker types will require longer.

Pasta verde is green pasta. The green varieties are made of spinach and durum semolina flour, enriched with egg yolks. Thus green pasta, which eliminates white flour, starch and salt, is less fattening. It is also more nutritious because of the spinach and egg yolks; it tastes delicious and looks beautiful when served. Tomato noodles are pale and become paler when cooked; the flavor is only a hint of tomato. This is a new type of pasta; it will be available eventually, although hard to find now.

HOW TO EAT PASTA

Italians believe that the way a man eats pasta will reveal his character and the place where he was born; whether he is a gastronome or a glutton, generous or miserly, honest or deceitful, stable or emotionally disturbed. The proper way to eat pasta is to use just the fork; push a small amount of the pasta away from you on the plate and neatly twirl it. "Don't disgrace the pasta with a spoon!" was what Papa Celli used to say. Not only in America but even in Italy one sees people tackling the pasta with fork and spoon. A novice may assume that is the proper way, but the restaurants who present spoons to eat pasta should take down their signs that say "Italian Cuisine" and change them to "Americanized Italian Food." If the pasta is sauced just right, it won't be swimming, but each strand will be delicately coated. (If you are more comfortable using a spoon, do so!)

PASTA PRIMAVERA I

TIME: 15 MINUTES
SERVINGS: 8
CALORIES: 235 PER SERVING OF PASTA, SAUCE AND CHEESE

1 *pound zucchini*
1 *pound fresh plum tomatoes*
4 *large fresh mushrooms*
3 *tablespoons vegetable oil*
6 *shallots, peeled*
6 *sprigs of Italian parsley*
2 *tablespoons minced fresh basil, or 1 tablespoon dried basil*
1 *small garlic clove, peeled*
1 *tablespoon Italian seasoning*
½ *cup chopped cooked broccoli*
   salt and pepper
1 *pound pasta (thin spaghetti, green spinach noodles, homemade pasta, or other very thin pasta)*
¼ *cup freshly grated Parmesan cheese*

Fill a large pot with water and start heating it for the pasta. Wash and trim zucchini, tomatoes and mushrooms, but do not peel. Pour the oil into a large skillet, but do not yet put the pan over heat. Dice unpeeled zucchini and tomatoes into the oil, then the shallots. Slice the mushrooms into the mixture and snip the leafy parts of the parsley into the mixture. Add the basil. Crush or purée the garlic into the pan, and add seasoning and cooked broccoli. Turn on the heat to medium-high and cook, while stirring often with a wooden spoon. After 10 minutes, taste, and add salt and pepper to taste.

Add pasta and 1 tablespoon salt to rapidly boiling water and stir.

Use your own judgment as to when the sauce is ready, but it should be cooked in 8 to 10 minutes. If you want a smoother sauce, you can cook it longer, or even purée it, but best for the *primavera* is to have a slight texture in the vegetables, so that you can still chew them and identify each one. Check the pasta by pulling a strand out of the water and biting it to see if it has the right *al dente* for your taste; *don't overcook.* Pour small amounts of water out of the pot, then pour the pasta into a large strainer. Shake quickly and return to the pot while it is still hot.

Pour the sauce over the pasta, a small amount at a time, and toss with two forks to mix before adding more. Add half of the Parmesan cheese, and toss again. Taste, and add more salt and pepper if needed. Serve immediately in heated small soup dishes or pasta bowls. Serve remaining cheese in a separate bowl, to be added according to individual taste.

VARIATIONS ON PRIMAVERA SAUCE: Omit mushrooms or broccoli. Add chopped eggplant, green peppers, pine nuts, almonds or pimientos.

For a creamy texture, add ¼ cup skim-milk ricotta cheese during final moments of cooking the sauce.

PASTA AL SEGRETO

Prepare sauce for pasta. Cook the pasta until less than *al dente*, actually slightly undercooked. Use a skillet large enough to hold the pasta. Place skillet over low to medium heat and add just enough oil to keep the pasta from sticking. Heat until moderately hot. When the pasta is still a few minutes undercooked, drain it and add to the skillet. Add 1½ cups of prepared sauce, and mix and cook together, to develop the full taste of the sauce, for a few minutes. Add ¼ cup freshly grated Parmesan cheese, mix, and at once transfer to a large serving dish. Spoon remaining sauce over the top, and grind black pepper over all. This works well for Pasta Primavera, and you will note the method is suggested for other preparations as well.

PASTA PRIMAVERA II

TIME: 15 MINUTES
SERVINGS: 8
CALORIES: 235 PER SERVING OF PASTA, SAUCE AND CHEESE

       1 *pound zucchini*
       ½ *pound broccoli*
       ½ *pound fresh green beans*
       2 *tablespoons vegetable oil*
       6 *shallots, peeled*
       1 *garlic clove, peeled*
       ¼ *cup chopped fresh Italian parsley*
       2 *tablespoons minced fresh basil*
       1 *pound pasta*
          salt and pepper
       ¼ *cup freshly grated Parmesan cheese*

Fill a large pot with water and start heating it for the pasta. Wash and trim zucchini, but do not peel. Wash and trim broccoli and green beans. Chop all vegetables, still raw, into small pieces. Heat oil in a large skillet and add green vegetables. Chop shallots into the pan and push garlic through a press into the mixture. Cover and oil-steam for 5 minutes. Uncover, stir to mix well, and add parsley and basil. Cover again and continue to cook until vegetables are done to your taste; they should still be crunchy.

Meanwhile cook pasta until *al dente*. When sauce is ready, season with salt and pepper to taste. Toss with pasta and sprinkle with cheese.

VARIATIONS: The basic recipe gives an all-green sauce. If you like, add 4 fresh plum tomatoes, washed and chopped (about 1 cup), or 1 cup canned plum tomatoes, after cooking green vegetables for 5 minutes. If you use canned tomatoes, add very little liquid.

Add diced raw eggplant to cook with the green vegetables.

For a creamy sauce, add ¼ cup skim-milk ricotta cheese during final minutes of cooking the sauce.

LINGUINE WITH CAPER-ANCHOVY SAUCE

TIME: 10 MINUTES
SERVINGS: 8
CALORIES: 260 PER SERVING OF PASTA AND SAUCE

3 *anchovy fillets*
3 *tablespoons capers*
1 *garlic clove, peeled*
3 *tablespoons olive oil*
¼ *cup dry white wine*
¼ *cup chopped fresh Italian parsley*
   freshly ground black pepper
1 *pound linguine*
1 *tablespoon salt*

Fill a large pot with water and start heating it for the pasta. Make the sauce in a large pasta bowl. Mash anchovies and capers together, push garlic through a press into the mixture, and beat in the oil, 1 tablespoon at a time, to make a smooth paste. Mix in wine and parsley. Taste, and add as much black pepper as you like. When water is boiling, add linguine and salt and cook until *al dente*. Drain well, then turn pasta into the bowl of sauce and mix well.

VARIATION: Omit capers and white wine for a plain anchovy sauce.

LINGUINE ALLA LISA

TIME: 10 MINUTES
SERVINGS: 4
CALORIES: 275 PER SERVING OF PASTA AND SAUCE

2   tablespoons olive oil
2   garlic cloves, peeled
¼   teaspoon crushed red pepper
½   pound linguine
    salt

Fill a large pot with water and start heating it for the pasta. Heat olive oil in a large skillet and push garlic through a press into the oil. Add red pepper. Cook for a few minutes. Add linguine and ½ tablespoon salt to the rapidly boiling water, and cook until pasta is *al dente.* Drain, and turn into the oil and garlic. Toss to coat the pasta well and serve immediately.

VARIATION: Sprinkle pasta with grated Parmesan cheese.

LINGUINE WITH EGG AND BASIL SAUCE

TIME: 10 MINUTES
SERVINGS: 4
CALORIES: 272 PER SERVING OF PASTA AND SAUCE

2   eggs
½   pound linguine fine or capellini
½   tablespoon salt
⅓   cup chopped fresh basil
¼   cup grated pecorino cheese
    freshly ground black pepper

Fill a large pot with water and start heating it for the pasta. Beat the eggs. When water is boiling, add linguine and salt and cook until *al dente,* 4 or 5 minutes. Drain, then return to the still hot pot. Pour in the eggs and toss rapidly; the eggs will cook in the heat of the pasta. Add basil, cheese, and pepper to taste, toss quickly, and serve at once.

LINGUINE WITH NAPOLEON'S PASTA SAUCE

TIME: 15 TO 20 MINUTES
SERVINGS: 8
CALORIES: 325 PER SERVING OF PASTA AND SAUCE

> 2 *half-breasts of chicken, boneless and skinless, 5 ounces each*
> 4 *fresh plum tomatoes*
> ~~2 tablespoons unsalted butter~~ *cooking spray*
> 4 *shallots, peeled and minced*
> 3 *tablespoons chopped fresh Italian parsley*
> ¼ *cup chicken stock*
> ¼ *cup brandy*
> ¼ *teaspoon crumbled dried orégano*
>   *salt and pepper*
> 1 *pound linguine or fettuccine*

Fill a large pot with water and start heating it for the pasta. Flatten the chicken breasts and chop into small dice. Wash tomatoes, remove hard portion near stem, and chop; there should be ½ cup. Melt the butter in a large skillet and add shallots and part of the parsley. Sauté for a few minutes, then add chicken bits and toss until slightly browned. Add stock, cover the pan, and cook for a few minutes longer. Heat the brandy, pour it over the chicken, and ignite. When the flame dies out, stir, then add tomatoes, orégano, salt and pepper to taste, and remaining parsley. Cook for 5 minutes.

Meanwhile, when water is boiling add linguine or fettuccine and 1 tablespoon salt and cook until pasta is nearly done, still slightly undercooked. Drain pasta and add to the sauce in the skillet. Mix sauce and pasta quickly, then let everything cook together for a few minutes. (This is the *al segreto* method.) Serve at once, with Parmesan cheese if you like.

VARIATION: For a lighter sauce, omit brandy and substitute white wine.

PASTA "IL CLEMENTE"
Linguine with Three Cheeses

TIME: 10 TO 12 MINUTES
SERVINGS: 8
CALORIES: 325 PER SERVING OF PASTA AND SAUCE

  2 tablespoons olive oil
  1 garlic clove, peeled
  ¼ cup chopped fresh Italian parsley
  1 pound linguine
     salt
  ½ cup crushed Gorgonzola cheese
  ¼ cup grated Parmesan cheese
  ¼ cup grated pecorino cheese
     freshly ground black pepper

Fill a large pot with water and start heating it for the pasta. Heat the oil in
a large skillet and push the garlic through a press into the oil. Add part of
the parsley and sauté for a few minutes. Set aside until pasta is cooked. Add
linguine and 1 tablespoon salt to the rapidly boiling water and cook until *al
dente.* Drain pasta, transfer to the skillet with the garlic and oil, and toss. Add
the three kinds of cheese, a little at a time, and keep tossing until the entire
amount is mixed into the pasta. Cook for 3 minutes. Add pepper to taste, salt
if needed, and the rest of the parsley. Serve immediately.

PASTA WITH FENNEL AND BASIL SAUCE

TIME: 15 MINUTES
SERVINGS: 8
CALORIES: 255 PER SERVING OF PASTA, SAUCE AND CHEESE

  1 tablespoon vegetable oil
  1 tablespoon unsalted butter
  4 shallots, peeled
  ½ cup minced fresh fennel
  ⅓ cup chopped fresh Italian parsley
  3 large basil leaves
  1 pound thin pasta
  1 tablespoon salt
  3 tablespoons grated Parmesan cheese

Fill a large pot with water and start heating it for the pasta. Heat oil and
butter in a large skillet. Mince the shallots into the skillet, and add the fennel
and part of the parsley. Sauté for a few minutes, then add the rest of the
parsley and snip the basil into the mixture. Cook for 3 or 4 minutes, stirring
often with a wooden spoon to give a creamy texture. When the water is

rapidly boiling, add the pasta and salt and cook until *al dente*. Drain pasta, and turn into a serving bowl. Add the sauce and the grated cheese, toss to mix well, and serve immediately.

VARIATION: If you don't have fresh fennel, use 2 tablespoons fennel seeds, crushed lightly in a mortar.

Recently, dried wild fennel *(finocchio selvaggio)* has been available in Italian groceries. This would be excellent for this dish. Crush enough of the dried herb to have 2 tablespoons.

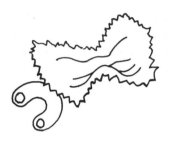

PASTA WITH RICOTTA ROMANA SAUCE

TIME: 10 MINUTES
SERVINGS: 4
CALORIES: 330 PER SERVING OF PASTA, SAUCE AND CHEESE

    ½ *pound fresh plum tomatoes*
    ½ *pound thin pasta (fine linguine or spaghettini)*
    ½ *tablespoon salt*
    2 *tablespoons olive oil*
    1 *garlic clove, peeled*
    3 *tablespoons minced fresh basil*
    ⅓ *cup minced fresh Italian parsley*
    ½ *cup chunks of skim-milk ricotta cheese*
    3 *tablespoons grated Parmesan cheese*

Fill a large pot with water and start heating it for the pasta. Wash tomatoes, remove hard portion near stem, and chop; there should be 1 cup. When water is rapidly boiling, add pasta and salt and cook for 4 to 5 minutes, until *al dente*. While pasta cooks, heat olive oil in a saucepan and push garlic through a press into the oil. Sauté for 1 minute, then add chopped tomatoes, basil and parsley. Cook until reduced to sauce consistency. Drain cooked pasta and return to the pot. Pour in tomato sauce, toss, then add ricotta and toss again. Sprinkle with Parmesan cheese and serve at once.

PASTA WITH ROASTED PEPPER SAUCE ALLA STELLA

TIME: 20 MINUTES
SERVINGS: 8
CALORIES: 270 PER SERVING OF PASTA AND SAUCE

2 *large red bell peppers*
2 *large green peppers*
1 *pound fresh plum tomatoes*
1 *onion, 2 ounces*
1 *pound thin pasta or pennine (quills)*
 salt
2 *tablespoons olive oil*
1 *garlic clove, peeled*
⅓ *cup chopped fresh Italian parsley*
 pepper

Roast the peppers over direct heat or under a broiler until the skin is browned. When they are cool enough to handle, peel off the skins; do not wash the peppers. (Washing removes the roasted flavor that gives the character to the sauce.) If some blackened specks of peel remain on the peppers, it doesn't matter, as they are edible. Discard ribs and seeds, and dice peppers. Wash tomatoes, discard hard portion near stem, and chop. Peel and mince the onion. Put tomatoes and peppers in a blender container, and reduce to a purée. Fill a large pot with water and start heating it for the pasta. When rapidly boiling, add pasta and 1 tablespoon salt and cook until *al dente;* the time depends on the pasta—thin spaghetti or thin linguine will need only 4 or 5 minutes; pennine may need a few minutes longer.

Heat oil in a deep saucepan and push garlic through a press into the oil. Add onion and sauté until onion is translucent. Add the pepper and tomato purée and the parsley and cook for 5 or 6 minutes. Season with salt and pepper to taste. Drain the pasta and serve with the sauce.

VARIATION: Combine pasta and sauce by the *al segreto* method. Undercook pasta, and turn into saucepan to finish cooking with the sauce for about 2 minutes.

PASTA CON SALSA ALLA NINO, IL CAMINETTO, NEW YORK CITY

TIME: 25 MINUTES
SERVINGS: 8
CALORIES: 300 PER SERVING OF PASTA, SAUCE AND CHEESE

½   *pound zucchini*
½   *pound fresh plum tomatoes*
4   *shallots*
1   *pound penne, ziti or shells*
1   *tablespoon salt*
1   *tablespoon vegetable oil*
¼   *pound lean beef, ground*
¼   *cup chopped fresh Italian parsley*
⅓   *teaspoon Italian seasoning*
1   *cup skim-milk ricotta cheese*
3   *tablespoons grated Parmesan cheese*

Fill a large pot with water and start heating it for the pasta. Wash and trim zucchini and chop, then mince; there should be 1 cup. Wash tomatoes, remove hard portion near stem, and chop; there should be 1 cup. Peel and mince shallots. When water is rapidly boiling, add pasta and salt and cook until *al dente,* or until as tender as you like. Heat oil in a large skillet and sauté shallots and beef until shallots are translucent and beef is no longer red, a few minutes. Add zucchini and sauté for 3 minutes; then add tomatoes, parsley and Italian seasoning, and cook for 10 minutes. Drain cooked pasta and turn into a pasta bowl with ricotta and Parmesan cheeses; toss well. Pour beef-zucchini sauce over and toss again. Accompany at table with more grated Parmesan cheese.

VARIATION: Undercook pasta and add to the sauce to finish cooking as in the *al segreto* method.

GREEN FETTUCCINE WITH RICOTTA SAUCE

TIME: 10 MINUTES
SERVINGS: 8
CALORIES: 260 PER SERVING OF PASTA AND SAUCE

  2 *cups skim-milk ricotta cheese*
  ½ *cup liquid skim milk*
  3 *tablespoons grated Parmesan cheese*
  ¼ *cup chopped fresh basil*
  3 *tablespoons chopped fresh Italian parsley*
  1 *pound green fettuccine*
  1 *tablespoon salt*

Fill a large pot with water and start heating it for the pasta. Mix ricotta with milk and Parmesan until the texture is smooth and creamy. Stir in the herbs. When water is boiling, add fettuccine and salt and cook until *al dente*. Drain, and turn into a large pasta bowl. Pour the ricotta sauce over, toss, and serve at once.

VARIATION: Heat ricotta sauce. Undercook pasta as for *al segreto* method. Drain and toss with 1 tablespoon butter, then turn into the ricotta sauce and cook for a few minutes. Serve with more grated cheese and freshly ground black pepper.

FETTUCCINE WITH RICOTTA-EGG SAUCE

TIME: 10 MINUTES
SERVINGS: 8
CALORIES: 260 PER SERVING OF PASTA AND SAUCE

  1 *cup skim-milk ricotta cheese*
  3 *tablespoons liquid skim milk*
  3 *tablespoons grated pecorino cheese*
  ⅓ *cup chopped fresh basil*
  2 *eggs*
  1 *pound fettuccine*
  1 *tablespoon salt*
     freshly ground black pepper

Fill a large pot with water and start heating it for the pasta. Mix ricotta, skim milk, pecorino cheese and basil. Beat the eggs lightly. When water is boiling rapidly, add fettuccine and salt and cook until the pasta is *al dente*. Drain well, then turn into a warmed pasta bowl. Pour in the eggs and toss rapidly; the eggs will cook in the heat of the pasta. Add the cheese mixture, toss again, and sprinkle with black pepper to taste.

FETTUCCINE WITH SALMON SAUCE ALLA BENNY

TIME: 15 MINUTES
SERVINGS: 8
CALORIES: 300 PER SERVING OF PASTA AND SAUCE

½ *pound dressed fresh salmon, without bones or skin*
½ *pound fresh plum tomatoes*
6 *to 8 shallots*
1 *pound fettuccine*
1 *tablespoon salt*
2 *tablespoons unsalted butter*
3 *tablespoons light cream*
   black pepper

Fill a large pot with water and start heating it for the pasta. Cut salmon into small pieces. Wash tomatoes, remove hard portion near stem, and chop; there should be 1 cup. Peel and mince shallots; there should be ⅓ cup. When water is rapidly boiling, add fettuccine and salt and cook until pasta is cooked *al dente*. Melt butter in a large skillet and sauté shallots until translucent. Add chopped tomatoes and cook for 5 minutes. Add salmon pieces and cream and cook over low heat for a few minutes, until salmon is cooked. Add pepper to taste. When pasta is cooked to taste, drain, and return to the warm pot. Turn salmon sauce into it, toss quickly, and serve at once.

VARIATION: Instead of fresh salmon, use ½ pound smoked salmon, cut into small pieces. Omit tomatoes from this version.

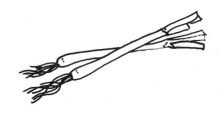

PASTA ALLA RUSSO
Egg Noodles with Caviar-Cream Sauce

TIME: 10 MINUTES
SERVINGS: 8
CALORIES: 265 PER SERVING WITH SOUR CREAM, 235 WITH RICOTTA

    1 cup sour cream or skim-milk ricotta cheese
    2 ounces caviar (of your choice)
    2 egg yolks, at room temperature
    1 tablespoon good Russian vodka
    ¼ cup grated Parmesan cheese
    3 sprigs of Italian parsley, snipped
    2 teaspoons snipped fresh chives
      black pepper
    1 tablespoon salt
    1 pound fresh thin egg noodles or fettuccine

Fill a large pot with water and start heating it for the pasta. Combine sour cream, or ricotta cheese, and caviar in a bowl and blend well. Add egg yolks, vodka and Parmesan cheese, and mix until smooth. Add herbs and freshly ground pepper to taste. (Salt is not needed, as caviar and Parmesan add enough salt.) Add 1 tablespoon salt and the pasta to the pot of rapidly boiling water and cook pasta for 4 or 5 minutes. Transfer pasta to a warm serving bowl. Add caviar-cream sauce and toss. Add more Parmesan cheese and freshly ground pepper if desired.

PASTA ALLA FRANCO
Spaghetti with Egg-Spinach Sauce

TIME: 10 MINUTES
SERVINGS: 8
CALORIES: 285 PER SERVING OF PASTA, SAUCE AND CHEESE

    1 pound fresh spinach
    4 egg yolks, well beaten
    3 sprigs of Italian parsley, chopped
    ½ teaspoon grated nutmeg
    ½ teaspoon white pepper
    1 tablespoon salt
    1 pound thin spaghetti
    ½ cup grated Parmesan cheese

Fill a large pot with water and start heating it for the pasta. Wash spinach carefully, remove any damaged leaves and all coarse stems, and drain. Chop spinach to small bits. Put raw spinach in a blender container with egg yolks, parsley, nutmeg and white pepper, and blend to a purée, like a paste. Add salt and pasta to the rapidly boiling water and cook pasta until done to your taste; 5 or 6 minutes is ample. Drain cooked pasta and transfer to a warm serving bowl. Add Parmesan cheese and the sauce, and toss well.

PASTA ALLA TOSCANA

TIME: 15 MINUTES
SERVINGS: 8
CALORIES: 340 PER SERVING OF PASTA AND SAUCE

> 1 tablespoon olive oil
> 1 tablespoon unsalted butter
> ⅓ cup chopped shallots
> ½ pound chicken livers, sliced
> 3 tablespoons dry white wine
> 1 pound thin pasta
> 1 tablespoon salt
> 4 eggs
> ¼ cup grated Parmesan cheese
> 3 tablespoons chopped fresh Italian parsley

Fill a large pot with water and start heating it for the pasta. Heat oil and butter in a skillet and sauté shallots in it until they are translucent. Add chicken livers and sauté, turning them often, until the slices are no longer pink inside. Add wine and cook for 2 minutes longer. Add the pasta and salt to the rapidly boiling water and cook for 6 minutes, until *al dente*. Beat the eggs with the cheese and parsley until smooth. Drain pasta and transfer to a large bowl. At once pour the egg mixture over pasta and mix thoroughly (the heat of the pasta will cook the eggs). Add the chicken-liver mixture and toss again. Serve with more cheese if you like.

PASTA WITH UNCOOKED FRESH TOMATO SAUCE

TIME: 10 MINUTES
SERVINGS: 8
CALORIES: 300 PER SERVING OF PASTA AND SAUCE

    1 *pound fresh tomatoes*
    2 *tablespoons vegetable oil*
    3 *small shallots, peeled and chopped*
  ½ *cup snipped fresh basil leaves*
    1 *garlic clove, peeled and crushed*
        salt and black pepper
    1 *pound pasta (egg noodles, fettuccine or thin spaghetti)*

Fill a large pot with water and start heating it for the pasta. Peel the tomatoes and remove hard portion at stem end. Cut into pieces and drop into a blender container. Add oil, shallots, basil leaves and garlic. Blend at high speed for 2 seconds. If the mixture is not puréed, whirl for a few seconds longer until it is. Add salt and freshly ground pepper to taste. When the water is boiling, add the pasta and 1 tablespoon salt and cook until done to your taste. Drain, and transfer to a serving bowl. Pour the sauce over the pasta, toss to mix, and taste; you may want to add more black pepper. (Usually cheese is not added to this sauce.) Serve at once.

VARIATION: Reserve the tomatoes until herbs are puréed. Add them, cut into dice, to the rest of the sauce just before serving for a chunky-style sauce.

PASTA WITH CLAMS AND OYSTERS

      TIME: 15 MINUTES
SERVINGS: 8
CALORIES: 285 PER SERVING OF PASTA AND SAUCE

  18 *fresh clams*
   8 *fresh oysters*
   2 *tablespoons olive oil*
   1 *garlic clove, peeled*
   1 *pound vermicelli*
   1 *tablespoon salt*
  ½ *cup dry white wine*
  ⅓ *cup chopped fresh Italian parsley*
   1 *tablespoon unsalted butter*

Scrub the clams, open them (see p. 248), and mince them (see Note, p. 98). Scrub oysters, open them, and mince, using the same method as for clams. There should be ½ cup of each kind of shellfish. Fill a large pot with water and start heating it for the pasta. Heat oil in a skillet and add the whole garlic clove. Sauté for a few minutes, then remove and discard garlic. When water is rapidly boiling, add vermicelli and salt and cook for 3 or 4 minutes, until just *al dente*. While pasta cooks add minced shellfish to the skillet with wine and parsley and cook over low heat for 5 minutes. Put the butter in a warmed large bowl. Drain pasta and toss in the buttered bowl. Pour in the sauce, mix thoroughly, and serve at once.

PASTA WITH WHITE MUSSEL SAUCE

TIME: 20 MINUTES
SERVINGS: 4
CALORIES: 355 PER SERVING OF PASTA AND SAUCE

        2 *dozen mussels*
        1 *tablespoon salt*
        ½ *pound linguine*
        2 *tablespoons vegetable oil*
        1 *garlic clove, peeled*
        3 *shallots, peeled*
        ½ *cup chopped fresh Italian parsley*
        ½ *cup dry white wine*
        3 *egg yolks*
        ¼ *cup freshly grated Parmesan cheese*
            freshly ground black pepper

Bring a large pot of water to a boil to cook the pasta. Scrub mussels with a stiff brush or plastic pot scrubber, and remove beards. Cover with cold water and soak for 5 minutes. Lift mussels from water and open them as you would open fresh clams. Do this over a bowl to save juices, and strain juices to remove any sand. Add salt and linguine to rapidly boiling water and cook while completing the sauce.

Heat the oil in a skillet. Push garlic through a press into the oil, dice the shallots into the oil, and add the parsley. Sauté all together for a few minutes. Put opened mussels and strained juices in a small saucepan and add the wine. Simmer for 5 minutes, then add mussels and liquid to the sautéed vegetables and cook for 1 or 2 minutes to mix well. Drain cooked pasta, add it to the sauce, and toss and heat for 1 minute. In a small bowl mix egg yolks and cheese until smooth. Pour over the pasta and cook all together for 1 more minute. Sprinkle with pepper and serve at once, with more cheese if you like.

PASTA WITH MUSSEL SAUCE CALABRIA ALLA JO

TIME: 20 MINUTES
SERVINGS: 8
CALORIES: 320 PER SERVING OF PASTA AND SAUCE

3½ *pounds mussels in shells*
½   *pound fresh plum tomatoes*
6   *to 8 shallots*
3   *tablespoons olive oil*
2   *garlic cloves, peeled*
¼   *cup chopped fresh Italian parsley*
2   *fresh basil leaves*
1   *pound thin pasta*
1   *tablespoon salt*

Scrub mussels with a stiff brush or plastic pot scrubber, and remove beards. Open the mussels in the same fashion as hardshell clams (see p. 248); do this over a bowl to save all the juices. Set mussels aside, and strain juices through a fine sieve lined with cheesecloth to get rid of any sand or bits of shell. Wash tomatoes, remove hard portion near stem, and chop; there should be 1 cup. Peel and chop shallots; there should be ⅓ cup. Fill a large pot with water and start heating it for the pasta. Heat the oil in a large skillet and push garlic through a press into the oil. Add shallots and half of the parsley, and snip basil leaves into the mixture. Sauté until shallots are translucent, then add mussels and strained juice and chopped tomatoes. Simmer over low heat for 6 minutes, until mussels are cooked; if you prefer, cook them for 8 minutes, but do not overcook, as this toughens them. Meanwhile, add pasta and salt to rapidly boiling water and cook until *al dente;* drain. Turn pasta into a large serving bowl, pour sauce over, and mix gently.

PASTA CON LE SARDE ALLA SICILIANA,
LA POSADA DA JOSE, PALERMO

We are presenting this recipe in the original style, although the cook may need to make some adjustments when marketing in the United States. We have no native fresh sardines like those of the Mediterranean, but fresh sardines are imported from Portugal and you may find them in some East Coast fish markets. Failing that, use small fresh herring. As a last resort use 2 cans (3¾ ounces each) imported boneless and skinless sardines. Instead of fresh wild fennel, with its more intense flavor, you will have to be satisfied with cultivated fennel.

TIME: 25 MINUTES
SERVINGS: 8
CALORIES: 350 PER SERVING OF PASTA AND SAUCE

1 pound fresh sardines
4 heads of wild fennel
1 white onion, 6 to 8 ounces
1 pound bucatini, penne or ziti
1 tablespoon salt
2 tablespoons olive oil
¼ cup dark raisins
2 tablespoons pine nuts (pignoli)
¼ cup minced fresh Italian parsley

Dress the sardines, removing bones, skins, heads and viscera. Cut the fish into small dice. Trim fennel, discard coarse outer ribs and top portions of inner ribs, and chop the hearts into very fine pieces. Peel and mince the onion. Fill a large pot with water, enough for the pasta, and bring to a boil. Add chopped fennel and boil for a few minutes, until soft. Use a skimmer or small strainer to transfer fennel pieces to several layers of paper towels to dry. Bring the water again to a boil and add pasta and salt. If you are using bucatini or ziti, break them into pieces. Cook pasta until cooked *al dente*, or as tender as you like; drain. Meanwhile heat the oil in a large skillet and sauté minced onion and fennel for a few minutes, until onion is translucent. Add diced sardines, the raisins and pine nuts, and continue to cook for about 10 minutes. Stir in the parsley. Pour the sauce over drained pasta. With this sauce do not add cheese.

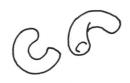

PASTA WITH PESTO SAUCE ALLA ELISA

TIME: 10 MINUTES
SERVINGS: 8
CALORIES: 290 PER SERVING OF PASTA AND SAUCE

1 cup chopped fresh basil
¼ cup chopped fresh Italian parsley
1 tablespoon crushed garlic
3 tablespoons olive oil
¼ cup skim-milk ricotta cheese
¼ cup grated Parmesan cheese
2 tablespoons grated pecorino cheese
   salt and pepper
1 pound very thin pasta (capellini preferred)

Fill a large pot with water and start heating it for the pasta. Put the basil in a blender container with parsley and garlic. Blend for 2 seconds. Start adding the oil, ½ teaspoon at a time, and blend for 1 second after each addition. When all is blended, turn into a large mixing bowl and mix in the three cheeses until smooth. Add salt and pepper to taste.

Meanwhile, when water is boiling add the pasta and 1 tablespoon salt and cook until pasta is *al dente.* Lift the pasta to a colander. Add a few drops of the cooking water to the *pesto* sauce, mix, then turn the pasta into the sauce and toss.

The sauce alone can also be used for *risotto* or fish, and about 4 tablespoons of the sauce will provide 75 calories.

RIGATONI ALLA NORMA, HOTEL JOLLY, PALERMO

TIME: 20 TO 25 MINUTES
SERVINGS: 8
CALORIES: 275 PER SERVING OF PASTA, SAUCE AND CHEESE

1 eggplant, 1 ½ pounds
   salt
1 pound rigatoni
2 tablespoons olive oil
1 garlic clove, peeled
¼ cup minced fresh basil
¼ cup minced fresh Italian parsley
¼ cup grated pecorino cheese

Wash and trim eggplant, but do not peel it. Cut it lengthwise into halves, and soak in water to cover with 1 tablespoon salt per quart of water for 15 minutes. Drain, rinse, drain again, and pat dry. Cut unpeeled eggplant into very thin slices, then cut slices into ¼-inch strips. While eggplant is soaking, fill a large pot with water and start heating it for the pasta. When rapidly boiling, add rigatoni and 1 tablespoon salt and cook for 10 minutes, or until done to your taste. While pasta cooks, heat the oil in a large skillet and push garlic through a press into the pan. Add eggplant strips and sauté them with the garlic, turning to cook all the pieces evenly. When rigatoni is cooked, drain and turn into a pasta bowl. Sprinkle with the herbs and cheese and toss to mix. Top with eggplant strips, toss again gently, and serve. Add more grated cheese if you like.

NOTE: In the original dish, the cheese used is *ricotta salata*. If you can find this salted, pressed ricotta, try it instead of pecorino.

SPAGHETTI ALLA CARBONARA I

TIME: 10 MINUTES
SERVINGS: 8
CALORIES: 300 PER SERVING OF PASTA AND SAUCE

1 tablespoon olive oil
1 garlic clove, peeled
3 tablespoons chopped lean bacon
½ cup dry white wine
3 eggs
¼ cup grated Parmesan cheese
¼ cup grated pecorino cheese
⅓ cup chopped fresh Italian parsley
1 pound very thin spaghetti
1 tablespoon salt

Fill a large pot with water and start heating it for the pasta. Heat oil in a very large skillet and drop in the whole garlic clove. When garlic is brown, remove it. Add chopped bacon and sauté until bacon is almost cooked. Add wine and cook for 2 minutes. Set aside. Beat eggs in a large bowl until well mixed, then stir in the cheeses and parsley. When water is boiling, add spaghetti and salt and cook for 4 or 5 minutes, until less than *al dente*. Drain spaghetti and toss it with the bacon mixture in the skillet over low heat. Add the egg and cheese mixture and toss rapidly so eggs will cook without scrambling. Add more cheese if you like, and serve at once.

SPAGHETTI ALLA CARBONARA II

TIME: 10 MINUTES
SERVINGS: 8
CALORIES: 310 PER SERVING OF PASTA AND SAUCE

- 1 tablespoon olive oil
- ¼ cup chopped shallots
- 3 tablespoons chopped prosciutto
- ½ cup dry white wine
- 3 eggs
- ⅓ cup grated Parmesan cheese
- ⅓ cup grated pecorino cheese
- ¼ cup chopped fresh Italian parsley
- 1 pound thin spaghetti
- 1 tablespoon salt

Fill a large pot with water and start heating it for the pasta. Heat oil in a very large skillet and sauté shallots with prosciutto until shallots are tender. Add wine and cook for 2 minutes. Beat eggs in a large bowl until well mixed, then stir in half of both cheeses and the parsley. When water is boiling, add spaghetti and salt and cook for 4 or 5 minutes, until less than *al dente*. Drain spaghetti and toss it with the mixture in the skillet over low heat. Add egg mixture and toss rapidly. Add the rest of the cheese, mix, and serve at once.

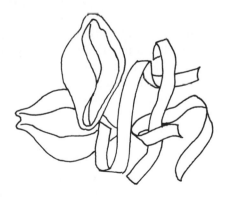

ROLLATINE DI MELANZANO, SEA PALACE, TAORMINA
Eggplant Rolls Filled with Pasta

TIME: 25 TO 30 MINUTES
SERVINGS: ABOUT 48 ROLLS
CALORIES: 50 PER ROLL

2 eggplants, 1 ½ pounds each
   salt
1 pound fresh plum tomatoes
3 tablespoons vegetable oil
1 pound thin spaghetti
1 garlic clove, peeled
⅓ cup chopped fresh Italian parsley
⅓ teaspoon Italian seasoning
   oil for baking pans
6 tablespoons grated Parmesan cheese

Wash and trim eggplants, and cut them into ¼-inch-thick slices. If eggplants are long and thin, cut slices at an angle to have a larger surface; fatter eggplants will give wide enough slices. Soak slices in cold water with 1 tablespoon salt per quart of water for 10 minutes. Drain the slices, rinse, and pat dry with paper towels. While eggplant is soaking, wash tomatoes, remove hard portion near stem, and chop; there should be 2 cups. Fill a large pot with water and start heating it for the spaghetti. Heat oil in a large skillet and sauté eggplant slices over brisk heat until just golden. If you need more oil, add it, ½ tablespoon at a time, but if the skillet is hot and eggplant slices well dried, more oil should not be necessary. Let oil drain back into the pan from sautéed eggplant slices, and place them on paper towels to drain well. When water is rapidly boiling, add thin spaghetti and 1 tablespoon salt and cook for 4 or 5 minutes, until cooked *al dente.* Drain pasta and return to the pot.

Reheat the oil remaining in the skillet. Push garlic through a press into the oil and sauté for a few minutes. Add chopped tomatoes and cook over low heat for 6 minutes. Add parsley and Italian seasoning and cook for another minute. Turn drained spaghetti into the skillet and mix well with the tomato sauce. Have ready 2 large shallow baking dishes, 7 by 13 inches or a similar size, and oil them lightly. Use a slotted spoon to place about 2½ tablespoons spaghetti on each eggplant slice. If possible, roll up the slices; if this is difficult, fold over the top part of each slice, then fold the bottom part over that, and fasten with a wooden food pick or small stainless-steel skewer. Place the rolls, seam side down, in the baking pans. Spoon any remaining sauce over the top, and sprinkle the cheese over all. Bake in a 350°F. oven for 10 minutes.

MACARONI MISTO

This recipe is ideal for using up an assortment of leftovers.

TIME: 25 MINUTES
SERVINGS: 10
CALORIES: 250 TO 300 PER SERVING, DEPENDING ON CHOICE OF MEAT,
            VEGETABLE AND SAUCE

 1 *pound pasta (penne, ziti, elbows, shells)*
 1 *tablespoon salt*
 1 *large green pepper*
 1 *onion, 3 ounces*
 2 *tablespoons vegetable oil*
 1 *garlic clove, peeled*
 2 *celery ribs, chopped*
 ½ *cup chopped cooked vegetables*
 ¼ *cup chopped olives*
 ¼ *cup chopped fresh Italian parsley*
 1 *cup chopped cooked meat (beef, chicken or ham), or seafood*
 ⅓ *teaspoon Italian seasoning*
 1 *cup sauce (tomato, cheese, wine, etc.)*
 ¼ *cup grated Parmesan cheese*

Fill a large pot with water and bring to a boil. Add pasta and salt and cook until pasta is *al dente;* do not overcook; the exact time will be determined by the kind of pasta. While pasta cooks, make the sauce. Wash and trim green pepper, discard ribs and seeds, and chop pepper. Peel and chop onion; there should be ½ cup. Heat the oil in a large saucepan and push the garlic through a press into the oil. Add onion, green pepper and celery, and cook for a few minutes, until onion is translucent. Add cooked vegetables, olives, parsley, meat and seasoning; cook until well mixed and hot, then add the sauce and simmer for a few minutes longer.

When pasta is cooked, drain and turn into a 2-quart casserole; whether round, square or rectangular does not matter. Pour the sauce mixture over and mix gently but thoroughly with wooden spoons. Sprinkle the cheese over the top. Bake in a preheated 350°F. oven for 8 to 10 minutes, or until cooked to your taste; the cheese topping should be golden.

PASTA AND SALMON SALAD SALADINO

TIME: 15 MINUTES
SERVINGS: 4
CALORIES: 225 PER SERVING

*1 cup chopped or flaked cooked fresh salmon, or canned salmon,
   or other cooked seafood*
⅓ cup chopped celery
⅓ cup chopped fresh Italian parsley
8 to 10 shallots, peeled and minced
¼ cup chopped pimiento
1 cup cooked pasta (elbows, ziti, penne or pieces of spaghetti)
2 tablespoons vegetable oil
*   juice of 1 lemon*
⅓ teaspoon dry mustard
¼ cup chopped fresh dill
*   salt and pepper*

Put fish in a large bowl and add celery, parsley, shallots and pimiento; mix. Add pasta and toss gently. Mix oil, lemon juice and mustard in a cup until mustard is dissolved. Mix in dill and pour sauce over fish and pasta. Add salt and pepper to taste if necessary. Chill for a few minutes before serving.

VARIATIONS: Add chopped olives, green peppers, tomatoes or hard-cooked eggs; or substitute any of these for one of the other ingredients.

Many different kinds of seafood can be used, even canned tuna; also various kinds of crustaceans. Try shrimps, mussels, clams, small squid, lobster, or use a mixture of several kinds.

LASAGNE

The lasagna noodle is different from all the other flat ribbon noodles listed in the introduction to this chapter, and not only because it is wider. Other noodles can be cooked and served in a tangle, but the lasagna noodle is always used flat. Because these noodles have to be arranged for the dish, it's especially important not to overcook them, lest they shred or break apart. When they are cooked just *al dente,* no further, remove pot from heat and carefully spread noodles out flat, one lasagna at a time, on a towel. Have ready a bowl of cold water and dip your hands into it as you handle the noodles; they will be hot.

VEGETARIAN LASAGNE BRUNO

TIME: 30 MINUTES
SERVINGS: 8
CALORIES: 315 PER SERVING

>   *1 pound green lasagna noodles*
>   *salt*
>   *1 pound fresh plum tomatoes*
>   *½ pound zucchini*
>   *½ pound eggplant*
>   *1 onion, 2 ounces*
>   *1 large green pepper*
>   *3 tablespoons vegetable oil*
>   *1 garlic clove, peeled*
>   *½ teaspoon Italian seasoning*
>   *½ teaspoon crushed red pepper*
>   *½ cup grated Parmesan cheese*

Fill a large pot with water and bring to a boil. Add 1 tablespoon salt and put in the noodles, one or two at a time so the water does not stop boiling. Cook the noodles until slightly less than *al dente,* then remove from heat and carefully arrange them on a towel. While noodles cook, prepare vegetables. Wash tomatoes, remove hard portion near stem, and chop; there should be 2 cups. Wash and trim zucchini and eggplant, and dice; there should be 1 cup of each. Peel and mince onion; there should be ¼ cup. Wash and trim pepper, discard ribs and seeds, and chop pepper. Heat the oil in a large skillet and push garlic through a press into the oil. Add zucchini, eggplant, onion and pepper and sauté, stirring a few times, for 5 minutes. Add tomatoes, Italian seasoning and red pepper, and cook for 10 minutes. Season with salt if needed.

Spoon a little sauce in the bottom of a 2-quart lasagne dish, and arrange a layer of lasagna on top. Spoon some sauce over. Continue with more layers of noodles and sauce until the dish is filled. Sprinkle cheese over the top. Bake in a preheated 350°F. oven for 8 to 10 minutes, or until the dish is baked to your taste.

LASAGNE WITH RICOTTA-MEAT SAUCE ALLA FODOR

TIME: 25 MINUTES
SERVINGS: 8
CALORIES: 335 PER SERVING

1 pound lasagna noodles
1 tablespoon salt
½ pound fresh plum tomatoes
10 to 12 shallots
2 tablespoons vegetable oil
1 garlic clove, peeled
½ pound lean beef, lamb or veal, ground
¼ cup chopped fresh Italian parsley
1 cup skim-milk ricotta cheese

Fill a large pot with water and bring to a boil. Add the salt and put in the noodles, one or two at a time so the water does not stop boiling. Cook noodles until slightly less than *al dente,* then remove from heat and carefully arrange them on a towel. While noodles cook, prepare the sauce. Wash tomatoes, remove hard portion near stem, and chop; there should be 1 cup. Peel and mince shallots; there should be ½ cup. Heat oil in a large skillet and push garlic through a press into the oil. Add shallots and sauté until translucent. Add ground meat and parsley and sauté until meat is no longer pink, a few minutes. Stir in tomatoes and cook for 8 minutes. If necessary add more seasoning to taste.

Use a flat 2-quart lasagna dish. Spoon a thin layer of sauce in the pan, then arrange a layer of noodles, another layer of sauce, and about half of the ricotta. Make a second layer of noodles, sauce and ricotta, and finish with the rest of the sauce. Bake in a preheated 350°F. oven for 8 to 10 minutes, or until done to your taste. Let set for a few minutes, then cut into squares to serve.

LASAGNE ALLA MADDALENA

TIME: 25 MINUTES
SERVINGS: 4
CALORIES: 260 PER SERVING

     5 *green lasagna noodles*
     2 *teaspoons salt*
     2 *bunches of scallions (18 scallions, no thicker than a pencil)*
     1 *pound zucchini*
     2 *cups canned peeled plum tomatoes*
  1 ½ *tablespoons vegetable oil*
     1 *teaspoon honey*
       oil for baking dish
     4 *ounces shredded skim-milk mozzarella cheese (1 cup)*

Fill a large pot with water and bring to a boil. Break each noodle into 2 pieces and drop them into the boiling water with 1 teaspoon salt. Cook until slightly less than *al dente,* then remove from heat and carefully place them on a towel. Wash and trim scallions and cut into pieces no thicker than ½ inch. Wash and trim zucchini and shred through a food grinder, using a plate with medium-size holes. Put the tomatoes through a food mill, making a thin purée. Heat the oil in a skillet and sauté scallions until tender. Add shredded zucchini and tomato purée and simmer for about 5 minutes, until zucchini is tender and sauce somewhat reduced. Stir in remaining salt and the honey. Oil a square 4-cup baking dish that is about 5 inches across. Arrange 2 pieces of lasagna on the bottom; they should just fit it neatly. Spoon in some sauce, then a few tablespoons of cheese. Continue to make layers, each time using 2 pieces of lasagna, a little sauce and a few tablespoons of cheese. Finish with cheese. There may be sauce left over; it can be refrigerated and used for another recipe. Cover the dish with foil and bake in a preheated 350°F. oven for 10 minutes, or until done to your taste. Serve from the dish.

TIMBALLO

A *timballo* is a dish similar to lasagne, but it is made in a round baking dish and cut into wedges like a pie. Usually it has many more layers than lasagne, and is much higher. In Italy the noodles are usually made at home *(pasta fresca)* and they are very thin and tender. The Italian lasagna noodles are the closest approximation to the homemade product.

Instead of using noodles, make the *timballo* with vegetable pancakes (see Zucchini Pancakes, p. 38) layered with the sauce or filling; or use very thin egg-cheese *frittatas.*

TIMBALLO ADELAIDE
Lasagne with Spinach and Cheese

TIME: 30 MINUTES
SERVINGS: 8
CALORIES: 350 PER SERVING

1 pound lasagna noodles
1 tablespoon salt
1½ pounds fresh spinach
1 pound fresh plum tomatoes
8 fresh mushrooms
8 to 10 shallots
2 tablespoons vegetable oil
¼ cup chopped fresh Italian parsley
⅓ teaspoon Italian seasoning
⅓ teaspoon grated nutmeg
1 cup skim-milk ricotta cheese
½ cup grated Parmesan cheese
½ cup shredded skim-milk mozzarella cheese

Fill a large pot with water and bring to a boil. Add the salt and put in the noodles, one or two at a time so the water does not stop boiling. Cook noodles until slightly less than *al dente,* then carefully drain them and arrange them on a towel. While noodles cook, prepare the sauce. Wash spinach thoroughly, then cook in just the water clinging to the leaves for about 4 minutes. Lift from the saucepan to a colander and chop; there should be 2 cups. Wash tomatoes, remove hard portion near stem, and chop; there should be 2 cups. Wash and trim mushrooms and chop; there should be ½ cup. Peel and mince shallots; there should be ⅓ cup. Heat oil in a large skillet and sauté shallots and mushrooms until shallots are translucent. Add spinach, parsley, Italian seasoning and nutmeg and continue to sauté for 2 minutes; then add tomatoes and simmer, stirring often to mix well, for 5 minutes.

Use a deep 2-quart round baking dish. Spoon a thin layer of spinach sauce in the bottom, then add a layer of noodles, another layer of spinach sauce, then about ¼ cup of the ricotta cheese and 2 tablespoons of Parmesan. Continue in the same way, making 5 layers of noodles and sauce and 4 layers of the cheeses. Top the last layer of noodles and sauce with the mozzarella. Bake in a preheated 350°F. oven for 8 to 10 minutes, or until done to your taste. Let the dish set and cool before cutting it into wedges.

TIMBALLO MISTO
Lasagne with Mixed Vegetables and Seafood

TIME: 25 MINUTES, EXCLUDING TIME TO COOK VEGETABLES AND
        SEAFOOD
SERVINGS: 8
CALORIES: 320 PER SERVING

    1 *pound lasagna noodles*
    1 *tablespoon salt*
   10 *to 12 shallots*
    2 *tablespoons vegetable oil*
    2 *cups chopped cooked vegetables*
    2 *cups Tomato Sauce (p. 245)*
    ⅓ *cup chopped fresh Italian parsley*
    1 *cup chopped cooked seafood*

VEGETABLES: Use your choice of broccoli, eggplant, spinach or zucchini. Blanch the vegetable until just barely tender, still a little crunchy. Or steam over water or oil-steam vegetable (see Broccoli all'Olio, p. 199). Vegetable can be chopped before or after cooking.

SEAFOOD: Use your choice of clams, crab meat, lobster, mussels or shrimps. Clams or mussels can be used raw or steamed. Crab, lobster or shrimps should be steamed or poached very briefly.

Fill a large pot with water and bring to a boil. Add the salt and put in the noodles, one or two at a time, so the water does not stop boiling. Cook noodles until slightly less than *al dente,* then carefully drain them and arrange them on a towel. While noodles cook, prepare the sauce. Peel and chop shallots; there should be ½ cup. Heat oil in a large skillet and sauté shallots until translucent. Add chopped vegetables and sauté for a few minutes longer. Add tomato sauce and parsley and simmer for 5 minutes. Add seafood and simmer and stir until sauce is well mixed and seafood hot.

Use a deep 2-quart round baking dish. Spoon a thin layer of sauce in the bottom, then add a layer of noodles. Continue to layer sauce and noodles, making 3 to 5 layers of each, ending with sauce. Bake in a preheated 350°F. oven for 8 to 10 minutes, or until done to your taste. Let the dish set and cool before cutting it into wedges.

TIMBALLO ALLA SILVESTRO
Lasagne with Chicken-Tomato Sauce

TIME: 30 MINUTES
SERVINGS: 12
CALORIES: 310 PER SERVING

1 ½ pounds lasagna noodles
      salt
1 pound fresh plum tomatoes
8 fresh mushrooms
1 onion, 2 ounces
1 large green pepper
2 tablespoons vegetable oil
⅓ cup chopped fresh Italian parsley
2 cups diced cooked chicken
⅓ teaspoon Italian seasoning
½ cup grated Parmesan cheese

Fill a very large pot with water and bring to a boil. Add 1½ tablespoons salt
and put in the noodles, one or two at a time so the water does not stop boiling.
Cook noodles until slightly less than *al dente,* then remove from heat and
carefully arrange them on a towel. While noodles cook, prepare the sauce.
Wash tomatoes, remove hard portion near stem, and chop; there should be
2 cups. Wash and trim mushrooms, and chop; there should be ½ cup. Peel
and mince onion; there should be ¼ cup. Wash and trim pepper, discard ribs
and seeds, and chop pepper. Heat oil in a large skillet and in it sauté onion,
mushrooms, green pepper and half of the parsley until onion is translucent
and green pepper soft. Add chicken and continue to sauté for a few minutes,
until chicken is lightly browned. Add tomatoes and Italian seasoning and
cook for about 10 minutes.

Use a deep 3-quart round baking dish. Spoon a thin layer of sauce in
the bottom, then add a layer of noodles. (You may need to trim noodles to
fit them into the round pan.) Spoon sauce over noodles, then sprinkle on
some Parmesan cheese. Continue making layers until you have about 5 layers
of noodles and 5 layers of sauce. Top with the rest of the sauce and cheese.
Bake in a preheated 350°F. oven for 8 to 10 minutes, or until done to your
taste. Let the dish set and cool before cutting it into wedges. Sprinkle remaining parsley around the edge. This is an excellent dish for buffet service.

TIMBALLO DI JOSEPH
Macaroni Pie

TIME: 30 MINUTES, EXCLUDING TIME FOR SOAKING MUSHROOMS
SERVINGS: 8
CALORIES: 365 PER SERVING

- ½ cup dried black mushrooms (about 1 ounce)
- 6 to 8 shallots
- 2 tablespoons vegetable oil
- ½ pound lean veal, ground
- ⅓ teaspoon Italian seasoning
- ¼ cup dry red wine
- ¼ pound fresh chicken livers
- 1 tablespoon salt
- 1 pound penne or pennine (quills)
- 2 eggs
- 3 tablespoons grated Parmesan cheese
- 3 tablespoons minced fresh Italian parsley
     black pepper
- ½ cup shredded skim-milk mozzarella

Rinse mushrooms and soak in water to cover for at least 30 minutes. Drain mushrooms and cut them into small pieces. (Any remaining soaking liquid can be strained through a cloth-lined sieve and reserved for later use.) Fill a large pot with water and start heating it for the pasta. Peel and chop shallots; there should be ⅓ cup. Heat oil in a large skillet, add shallots, and sauté until translucent. Stir in the veal, mushrooms and Italian seasoning, and sauté for about 5 minutes. Add wine and chicken livers and continue to cook, mixing and mashing as you do so livers and veal are well blended with vegetables. Livers and veal should not be overcooked. (If the texture becomes too dry, add some of strained mushroom soaking liquid.)

When water is boiling, add the salt and the penne or pennine and cook for 8 minutes, or until *al dente.* Do not overcook pasta, as it will be cooked further. Beat the eggs with Parmesan cheese and parsley. When pasta is done to your taste, drain in a colander, return to the pot, and at once add the egg mixture. Mix thoroughly. Pour veal and mushroom sauce over, again mix thoroughly, and season with pepper to taste. Turn the whole mixture into a shallow round baking dish that will hold about 8 cups. Sprinkle shredded mozzarella over the top. Slide into a preheated 350°F. oven and bake for 5 to 8 minutes, until cheese is melting. Cool the *timballo* for a few minutes, then cut into pie-shaped pieces to serve. Use for pasta course or for a main course.

VARIATIONS: Simplify the sauce by using only veal or only chicken livers. Use tomato sauce instead of veal and mushroom sauce. Use other kinds of pasta in place of penne.

For buffet meals or other special occasions, this can be baked in rectangular pans, then cut into small squares to serve. It can even be used for a first course or for cocktail party food; for these purposes cut into very small squares.

A *timballo* can be made with Artichoke Sauce or Primavera Sauce or Ricotta Sauce (see Index). It can make a complete meal, with salad and fruit and cheese.

RICE DISHES

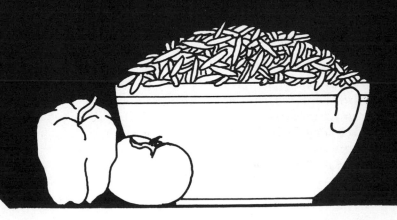

Riso is the word for uncooked grains of rice, but in food preparation it is often used interchangeably with *risotto,* the name for rice cooked with other ingredients. *Riso* when applied to cooked rice indicates just plain cooked rice with butter, no other additions.

While pasta is the universal starch throughout Italy, rice is the first choice in the North and is a strong second to pasta everywhere else. There are many famous variations of *risotto* prepared in the North. *Risotto* is served like pasta—as a first course or a main course, depending on the ingredients or sauce.

Just as a good brand of Italian pasta is essential for perfect results, so is good rice. It is tempting to say that you should use the fine rice from Italy exclusively, but it is not available everywhere. There are good American brands, however, that are easy to digest and nutritious. What is important is to use a rice that holds its firmness, that cooks *al dente* and does not cook to mush.

All the rice eaters of the world do not have the same notion of the perfect rice dish. Let us just think of rice Italian style—every kernel separate, good flavor, a recognizable texture—this is a preparation that one can enjoy on its own, not just a blotter for the sauce. There are probably 500 variations of *risotto*—vegetable creations; rice with seafood, meat, just herbs; *risotto* with Champagne (a dish prepared in Taormina); *risotto primavera* with shaved fresh zucchini. There are creamy, sweet, hot and spicy versions.

Risotto is an excellent dish for large dinner parties and for buffet meals. It doesn't need to be a hot dish; it also makes a great salad. Rice can be shaped or molded to enhance the presentation. These recipes are the merest sample of what you can do with this delicious grain.

RISOTTO

TIME: 20 MINUTES
SERVINGS: 6
CALORIES: 170 PER SERVING

   1 *tablespoon vegetable oil*
   1 *small onion, chopped*
   1 *cup uncooked natural brown rice or Arborio or Carolina rice*
   ¼ *cup dry Marsala wine*
   ½ *teaspoon Italian seasoning*
   2 *cups water*
   ¼ *cup grated Parmesan cheese*

Heat the oil in a deep saucepan, and sauté chopped onion in oil until translucent. Add rice and stir it to coat every kernel with oil. Add wine and Italian seasoning. Pour in ½ cup water and stir. Cover, and let the rice cook until the liquid is nearly absorbed, 4 to 6 minutes, then add remaining water. Cover again and cook for 10 minutes longer. Remove from heat and stir in the grated cheese just before serving. MAKES ABOUT 2½ CUPS.

VARIATIONS: When you start to sauté the onion, add garlic, chopped mushrooms or chopped green peppers or other vegetables.

Instead of water, chicken stock can be used to make a richer-tasting dish. It will also be more caloric.

The rice is *al dente* when cooked this long, but you may prefer it softer. If so, you may need to add a few tablespoons more water.

Instead of onion, use chopped shallots.

Instead of Marsala use dry white wine. Or omit wine altogether and add ¼ cup chopped fresh Italian parsley when adding Italian seasoning.

Tomatoes can be used for the liquid in place of water.

RISOTTO PIEMONTESE

TIME: 25 MINUTES, EXCLUDING TIME TO SOAK MUSHROOMS
SERVINGS: 8 (ABOUT ⅔ CUP)
CALORIES: 200 PER SERVING

½ cup dried black mushrooms (about 1 ounce)
½ cup dry Marsala wine
2 cups uncooked Italian rice
3 cups beef stock
2 tablespoons unsalted butter
3 tablespoons grated Parmesan cheese
¼ cup chopped fresh Italian parsley
⅓ teaspoon grated nutmeg
salt and pepper

Rinse mushrooms and soak in the Marsala for 30 minutes. Cut mushrooms into small pieces. Wash rice in cold water until water runs clear; drain well. Turn into a large saucepan and add beef stock, mushrooms and any remaining Marsala. Bring to a boil, cover, and simmer over low heat for 15 to 20 minutes, until *al dente*. Mix in butter, cheese, parsley, nutmeg, and salt and pepper to taste. Serve hot as a main dish, or as accompaniment to a meat dish.

VEGETABLE RISOTTO GIORGIO

TIME: 15 MINUTES, EXCLUDING TIME TO COOK RISOTTO
SERVINGS: 4
CALORIES: 190 PER SERVING

2 cups diced vegetables
3 tablespoons vegetable oil
4 shallots, peeled
1 garlic clove, peeled
3 tablespoons shredded fresh gingerroot
1 teaspoon Italian seasoning
4 sprigs of Italian parsley, chopped
1 cup cooked plain Risotto (p. 90), without cheese
    salt and pepper

VEGETABLES: Use any combinations of the following: asparagus, broccoli, eggplant, fennel, green beans, green peppers, mushrooms, okra, onions, pimientos, spinach, tomatoes, zucchini. Wash, peel, trim, according to the vegetable you are using, and cut into dice. Fennel and green beans should be blanched before adding. Other vegetables can be blanched if you prefer, but the steaming step cooks them adequately. Pour the oil into a large frying pan. Chop the shallots into the pan, and push the garlic through a press into the pan. Add gingerroot, Italian seasoning, parsley and vegetables. Cover, and steam with no added liquid. Stir often with a wooden spoon. (This "par-steaming" is a great way to cook vegetables.) When cooked to a nice bite, but not mushy, 8 minutes tops, uncover and gently stir in the *risotto*. Add salt and pepper to taste. Leave over heat just long enough for everything to be well mixed and hot, and serve at once.

VARIATIONS: Serve hot or cold as an unusual first course, or serve cold to accompany a main dish.

Mix cooked fish, chicken or veal with the *risotto* to make a main dish by itself.

Add ½ cup skim-milk ricotta or shredded skim-milk mozzarella, and spoon into a 4-cup casserole. Bake in a preheated 350°F. oven for 5 minutes, or until cooked to your taste.

Add 1 cup Tomato Sauce (p. 245), mix well, and spoon into a 4-cup casserole. Sprinkle ¼ cup grated Parmesan cheese on top, and bake in a 350°F. oven until cheese is golden.

RISOTTO PRIMAVERA ALLA RITA

TIME: 30 MINUTES
SERVINGS: 6
CALORIES: 250 PER SERVING

    1 zucchini, about 7 ounces
    ¼ pound fresh green beans
    6 to 8 shallots
    2 tablespoons unsalted butter
    1 cup uncooked Italian rice
    2 cups water
    ¼ cup chopped fresh basil
    ¼ cup chopped fresh Italian parsley
    ¼ cup grated Parmesan cheese

Wash and trim zucchini and cut into very thin long slivers, thinner than a match, like strings; there should be 1 cup. Wash and trim the green beans, blanch them until only slightly cooked, and drain. Cut beans into diagonal pieces. Peel and mince shallots; there should be ⅓ cup. Melt butter in a deep saucepan and sauté shallots until translucent. Add rice and turn it in the oil until all kernels are coated and beginning to look white. Add the water, cover the saucepan, and cook for 10 minutes. Uncover the pan and stir in zucchini strips, green beans, basil and parsley. Cover the pan again and cook for 10 minutes longer, until rice is *al dente.* Serve with the cheese.

MUSHROOM RISOTTO

TIME: 30 MINUTES
SERVINGS: 8
CALORIES: 210 PER SERVING

    ½ pound fresh mushrooms
    2 tablespoons unsalted butter
    ¼ cup chopped shallots
    ½ cup dry white wine
    2 cups uncooked Italian rice or natural brown rice
    5 cups chicken stock
    ¼ teaspoon Italian seasoning
    ½ cup minced fresh Italian parsley
       salt and pepper
    ¼ cup freshly grated Parmesan cheese

Wash and trim mushrooms, dry in paper towels, and slice; there should be 2 cups. Melt butter in a large saucepan, and add shallots and mushrooms. Sauté until shallots are translucent. Add white wine and continue to cook for 3 minutes. Add rice and stir, then add ½ cup of the stock and stir again. Cover and cook until the liquid is absorbed, then add another ½ cup stock, cover, and again cook until liquid is absorbed. Continue to add the stock, ½ cup at a time, and cook until absorbed, but keep checking the rice for the texture you want, as you may not want to add all of the stock. The texture of the rice should be *al dente,* not mushy or soupy. Stir in Italian seasoning, the parsley, and salt and pepper to taste. Just before serving stir in the cheese.

VARIATION: For a more intense mushroom flavor, use dried black mushrooms. Soak 1 cup (about 1¾ ounces dried) mushrooms in ½ cup dry Marsala for 30 minutes, or for less time if the cooking time will be lengthy. Do not use the stems, as they are tough and have less flavor than the caps. However, they can be used to flavor stock or soup where they are strained out. If any soaking liquid remains, strain through cloth and add to the recipe.

RISOTTO ALLA PRINCE STROZZI CON VERNACCIA

TIME: 30 MINUTES, EXCLUDING TIME FOR SOAKING MUSHROOMS
SERVINGS: 6
CALORIES: 215 PER SERVING

- ½ cup dried mushrooms (about 1 ounce)
- 6 to 8 shallots
- 1 tablespoon unsalted butter
- 2 tablespoons olive oil
- 1 cup uncooked Italian rice
- 2 cups dry white wine (Vernaccia preferred)
- 1 cup water
- ⅓ teaspoon Italian seasoning
- ¼ cup chopped fresh Italian parsley
- ¼ cup grated Parmesan cheese

Soak mushrooms in water for 30 minutes, or longer if you have time. Drain mushrooms and cut into small pieces. Peel and mince shallots; there should be ⅓ cup. Heat butter and oil in a deep saucepan. Add mushrooms and shallots and sauté until shallots are translucent. Add rice and turn it in the oil and butter until all kernels are coated and beginning to look white. Add wine, water and Italian seasoning, cover, and cook over low heat for 15 minutes. Uncover, add parsley, cover again, and cook until *al dente.* If rice becomes too dry before it is done to your taste, add more wine or water, 1 or 2 tablespoons at a time. Stir in cheese and serve.

RISOTTO WITH CHAMPAGNE ALLA BEPPE

TIME: 30 MINUTES, EXCLUDING TIME FOR SOAKING MUSHROOMS
SERVINGS: 6
CALORIES: 230 PER SERVING

  ½ cup dried mushrooms (about 1 ounce)
  6 to 8 shallots
  2 tablespoons unsalted butter
  1 cup uncooked Italian rice
  1 cup water
  2 cups dry Champagne
  ¼ cup chopped fresh Italian parsley
  2 basil leaves, minced
  ⅓ cup grated Parmesan cheese

Soak mushrooms in water for 30 minutes, or longer if you have time. Drain mushrooms, and cut into small pieces. Peel and mince shallots; there should be ⅓ cup. Melt butter and sauté shallots and mushrooms for a few minutes. Add rice, turn it over to coat all the grains with butter, and sauté for about 3 minutes. Add water and Champagne, cover, and cook over low heat for 10 minutes. Add herbs and half of the cheese and continue to cook for 10 to 15 minutes, until rice is cooked to your taste. Add remaining cheese when ready to serve.

RISOTTO WITH ARTICHOKES MARIO

TIME: 30 MINUTES, EXCLUDING TIME FOR COOKING ARTICHOKES
SERVINGS: 6
CALORIES: 210 PER SERVING

   2 *cooked large fresh artichoke bottoms (p. 195)*
   6 *to 8 shallots*
   2 *tablespoons olive oil*
   1 *cup uncooked Italian rice*
   2 *cups dry white Sicilian wine*
   1 *cup water*
   ¼ *cup chopped fresh Italian parsley*
   ⅓ *teaspoon crumbled dried orégano*
   ¼ *cup grated pecorino cheese*

When artichoke bottoms are cool enough to handle, remove all remaining leaves and the choke. Cut bottoms into small dice; there should be 1 cup. Peel and mince shallots; there should be ⅓ cup. Heat oil in a deep saucepan and add shallots and artichoke dice; sauté until shallots are translucent. Add rice and turn it in the oil until all kernels are coated and beginning to look white. Add wine and water, cover, and cook over low heat for 15 minutes. Uncover the saucepan, stir in parsley and orégano, cover again, and cook for 10 minutes longer, until liquid is all absorbed and rice is tender but not mushy. Stir in the cheese, or serve the cheese separately.

RICE WITH FRESH TOMATOES AND HERBS

TIME: 20 MINUTES
SERVINGS: 4
CALORIES: 250 WITH CHEESE, 220 WITHOUT CHEESE

   2 *tablespoons vegetable oil*
   2 *small shallots, peeled and diced*
   ¾ *cup uncooked natural brown rice*
   1 *pound ripe tomatoes*
  1½ *cups water*
   2 *teaspoons chopped fresh basil*
   ½ *teaspoon minced fresh sage*
   3 *tablespoons minced fresh Italian parsley*
   ¼ *teaspoon freshly ground pepper*
   ¼ *teaspoon salt*
   ¼ *cup grated Parmesan cheese (optional)*

Pour the oil into a saucepan and add the shallots; stir. Add uncooked rice and stir until all the grains are coated with oil. Peel the tomatoes and remove hard portion at stem end. Chop tomatoes.

(If you do not have ripe tomatoes, use 16 ounces canned peeled plum tomatoes. Pour off the juice into a 2-cup measure and add enough water to fill the measure. Chop the canned tomatoes.)

Add the water, chopped tomatoes, herbs and seasoning to rice. Cover and bring to a boil, then reduce to a simmer and cook for 15 minutes. Transfer to a warm bowl and add grated Parmesan cheese if desired.

VARIATIONS: Diced fresh mushrooms can be added to the rice.

Herbs can be varied; use orégano instead of sage, and fennel seeds in place of parsley. Or add a hot accent with cayenne pepper. If you are using some dried herbs, be sure to use at least 3 parts fresh herbs to 1 part dried herb.

RISOTTO WITH PROSCIUTTO AND MUSHROOMS

TIME: 25 MINUTES EXCLUDING TIME TO SOAK MUSHROOMS
SERVINGS: 8 (ABOUT ⅔ CUP)
CALORIES: 200 PER SERVING

½ cup dried black mushrooms (about 1 ounce)
½ cup dry Marsala wine
2 cups uncooked Italian rice
2 ounces prosciutto, chopped
3 cups water
1 tablespoon unsalted butter
⅓ cup chopped fresh Italian parsley
½ cup grated Parmesan cheese
  salt and pepper

Rinse mushrooms and soak in the Marsala for 30 minutes. Cut mushrooms into small pieces. Wash rice in cold water until water runs clear; drain well. Sauté prosciutto and mushrooms in a large saucepan over low heat for a few minutes. Add rice, water and any remaining Marsala. Bring to a boil, cover, and simmer over low heat for 15 to 20 minutes. When done as you like it, toss with butter, parsley and cheese, and season to taste.

VARIATION: Instead of dried mushrooms, use 1 small white truffle, cut into thin slices.

RISOTTO WITH CLAMS

TIME: 20 MINUTES
SERVINGS: 8 (ABOUT 1 CUP)
CALORIES: 260 PER SERVING

> 2 cups uncooked Italian rice
> 1 onion, 4 ounces
> 1 pound fresh plum tomatoes
> 2 tablespoons vegetable oil
> 1 cup chopped raw clams with natural juices
> ¼ cup dry red wine
> ¼ cup chopped fresh Italian parsley
>   black pepper

Wash rice in cold water until water runs clear; drain well. Peel and chop onion. Wash and peel tomatoes, and chop; there should be 2 cups. Heat the oil in a large saucepan and add chopped onion. Sauté until onion is translucent. Add the juice from the clams, the wine, rice and tomatoes. Mix well and bring to a boil. Cover, and simmer over low heat for 10 minutes. Stir in clams and parsley, and continue to cook until rice is done to your taste. Season with pepper; salt is probably not necessary, as clams are salty.

NOTE: To have 1 cup chopped clams, purchase about 3 dozen clams in the shell. Open them following the directions on page 248. Strain juices through a fine sieve to remove any sand, and chop clams on a board or put through a food grinder, using a plate with medium holes. Some markets may offer already shelled fresh clams, usually in pint containers. They must be refrigerated, and should be fresh, with clear juices.

VARIATION: Other varieties of seafood can be used—shrimps or mussels—alone or in a mixture with clams.

COLD RISOTTO RING

TIME: 20 MINUTES, EXCLUDING TIME TO MAKE RISOTTO
SERVINGS: 6
CALORIES: 120 PER SERVING

3 cups plain Risotto (p. 90), without cheese
2 green peppers
2 pimientos
5 very fresh mushrooms
   vegetable oil for mold
1 bunch of watercress
6 cherry tomatoes
6 pitted black olives

Make *risotto* and cool. Wash and trim peppers, discard ribs and seeds, and chop peppers. Rinse seeds from pimientos and chop them. Wash and trim mushrooms and slice or chop. Mix all these into *risotto,* and firmly press the mixture into a 4-cup ring mold that has been lightly oiled on the inside. Chill the mold for 10 minutes or longer if possible. Wash and dry watercress and separate leafy sprigs from stems. Wash cherry tomatoes and remove stems.

At serving time, dip mold into hot water. Place a round serving plate on top; holding plate and mold tightly together, flip over. Gently shake the mold to release the rice ring. Garnish the ring with cherry tomatoes and olives, and put the watercress sprigs in the center to make a leafy bouquet.

RISOTTO SALAD

TIME: 10 MINUTES, EXCLUDING TIME TO MAKE RISOTTO
SERVINGS: 6
CALORIES: 135 PER SERVING

3 cups plain Risotto (p. 90), without cheese
2 zucchini, 4 ounces each
¼ pound fresh plum tomatoes
10 pitted black olives
¼ cup chopped fresh Italian parsley
6 tablespoons Vinaigrette Dressing (p. 254)

Make *risotto* and cool. Wash and trim zucchini, and shred them. Wash tomatoes, remove hard portion near stem, and chop. Chop olives. Mix vegetables, olives and parsley into the rice and toss with the dressing. Serve in a large bowl, garnished with small lettuce leaves.

INSALATA DI RISO ALLA SAM

TIME: 25 MINUTES
SERVINGS: 8 (ABOUT 1 CUP)
CALORIES: 195 PER SERVING

2 cups uncooked Italian rice or natural brown rice
4 cups water
  salt
½ pound raw shrimps in shells
½ pound fresh plum tomatoes
2 small green peppers
3 shallots
¼ cup chopped fresh Italian parsley
2 tablespoons chopped fresh basil
3 tablespoons capers
2 hard-cooked eggs
6 pitted black olives
1 tablespoon olive oil
  juice of 1 lemon
  black pepper
6 parsley sprigs

Wash rice in cold water until water runs clear; drain well. Put 4 cups water and the rice in a large saucepan, and 1 teaspoon salt, or more salt if you prefer, and bring to a boil. Cover, and simmer over low heat for 15 to 20 minutes, until *al dente*. While rice cooks, shell and devein shrimps and poach them in water to cover for 5 minutes. Drain shrimps, cool, and chop. Prepare the vegetables: Wash tomatoes, cut out hard portion near stem, and chop; there should be 1 cup. Wash and trim green peppers, discard ribs and seeds, and cut peppers into thin slices. Peel and mince shallots. Put tomatoes, peppers, shallots, parsley, basil and capers in a large oval bowl. Shell eggs and cut into wedges or slices. Chop olives. Set eggs and olives aside for garnish. When shrimps are cooled and diced, add them to the vegetables. When rice is cooked, turn it into the bowl. Toss to mix well, then quickly toss with oil and lemon juice. Add more salt if needed, and black pepper to taste. Garnish the salad with egg pieces, chopped olives and parsley sprigs. Serve as salad or luncheon main course. Fabulous for buffet parties.

VARIATIONS: Use other vegetables. Use other seafood or more seafood. Add a small amount of mayonnaise to the dressing.

FISH, SHELLFISH
AND
CRUSTACEANS

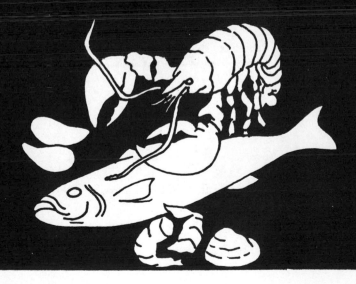

Italy is surrounded by the sea except in the North, and in that region there are large lakes and rivers. As a natural consequence fish and seafood are an important part of the Italian diet. Along the Adriatic, Ionian, Tyrrhenian and Ligurian seas fresh fish is easily available, and is purchased each morning for the day's meals.

While some fish in these waters and in the larger Mediterranean are not found in the Western Atlantic or along our Pacific Coast, good substitutions are easy to find. In America cod, flounders, halibut, salmon, snappers, striped bass and trout can be found in local fish markets and even in supermarkets. Also plentiful are clams, mussels, shrimps, squid and various crabs and lobsters.

For a healthful diet eat fish as often as possible. Fresh fish is delicious; it has as much protein as most meats, weight for weight, but is low in calories and low in the saturated fatty acids that lead to an increase in serum cholesterol. Only a few fish are "fatty," and even that varies with the season and life cycle of the fish.

Another plus is that fish can be simply and *quickly* prepared. A typical flounder fillet will be cooked in minutes, and even thicker fillets and whole fish need little more time. By varying the flavoring ingredients, you can prepare many different dishes with the same basic cooking technique. Of course fish, particularly sole and turbot, are the basis for elaborate preparations by famous chefs, but those dishes often seem to emphasize the sauce and garnish more than the fish. You will find nothing complicated here, because the emphasis is on recipes that will enhance the main ingredient and help you enjoy the natural taste of good fish and shellfish. You will find no recipes for fried fish here! Unfortunately many restaurants in the United States serve only fried fish. To fry a beautiful fresh fish to the point of being dry and tasteless is utterly wasteful. You must taste the freshness of the fish, properly prepared, delicately cooked, not the bread crumbs or the sauce.

Some of the recipes in this chapter are classic dishes that can be found throughout Italy. Others are dishes invented for this book, and a few are the creations of special friends who are professionals and epicures.

BAKED CODFISH VINCENZO

TIME: 15 TO 20 MINUTES
SERVINGS: 6
CALORIES: 185 PER SERVING

6 *fresh cod steaks, 5 or 6 ounces each*
½ *pound fresh plum tomatoes*
2 *tablespoons vegetable oil*
1 *onion, 3 ounces, peeled*
2 *potatoes, 3 ounces each, peeled*
¼ *cup chopped fresh Italian parsley*
¼ *cup tomato paste*
1 *bay leaf*
¼ *teaspoon Italian seasoning*
  salt and pepper

Rinse codfish and pat dry. Wash tomatoes, remove hard portion near stem, and chop; there should be 1 cup. Heat oil in a large skillet and chop onion and potatoes into the oil. Add half of the parsley and sauté for 2 minutes. Place codfish steaks on the vegetables, and pour in the tomatoes and tomato paste. Place bay leaf in the middle, and sprinkle the fish with Italian seasoning and salt and pepper to taste. Cover and cook over low heat for 10 minutes. Add the rest of the parsley for the last minute. Remove bay leaf and serve.

CODFISH IN WHITE-WINE SAUCE

TIME: 20 MINUTES
SERVINGS: 6
CALORIES: 145 PER SERVING

6 *pieces of boneless fresh cod, 4 ounces each*
1 *tablespoon unsalted butter*
1 *tablespoon vegetable oil*
4 *shallots, peeled*
½ *cup dry white wine*
½ *teaspoon salt*
¼ *teaspoon white pepper*
¼ *cup chopped fresh Italian parsley*
⅓ *cup seedless white grapes*

Rinse codfish and pat dry. Melt butter with oil in a large skillet. Mince shallots into the pan and sauté until they are translucent. Place cod pieces in the pan and pour in the wine. Sprinkle fish with salt, pepper and parsley, cover the skillet, and cook for 10 minutes. While fish is cooking, wash grapes and roll in a towel to dry. With a sharp knife cut each grape into 4 pieces. Add them to the fish, cover the pan again, and cook for 3 minutes longer.

CODFISH ADELAIDE

TIME: 20 MINUTES
SERVINGS: 6
CALORIES: 170 PER SERVING

6 *pieces of boneless fresh cod, 4 ounces each*
½ *pound fresh plum tomatoes*
2 *tablespoons vegetable oil*
1 *onion, 3 ounces, peeled*
¼ *cup chopped fresh Italian parsley*
⅓ *cup dark raisins*
¼ *cup tomato paste*
  salt and pepper

Rinse codfish and pat dry. Wash tomatoes, remove hard portion near stem, and chop; there should be 1 cup. Heat oil in a large skillet. Chop onion into the oil and sauté until translucent. Place fish pieces in the pan and sauté for a few minutes. Add parsley, raisins, tomatoes and tomato paste. Cover and cook for 10 minutes. Season with salt and pepper to taste.

CODFISH FRANCO
with Tomatoes and Caper Sauce

TIME: 15 MINUTES
SERVINGS: 6
CALORIES: 160 PER SERVING

6 *fresh cod steaks, 5 or 6 ounces each*
½ *pound fresh plum tomatoes*
2 *tablespoons vegetable oil*
1 *onion, 3 ounces, peeled*
3 *tablespoons capers*
6 *pitted black olives, chopped*
  salt and pepper
6 *tablespoons chopped fresh Italian parsley*

Rinse codfish and pat dry. Wash tomatoes, remove hard portion near stem, and chop; there should be 1 cup. Heat oil in a large skillet. Chop onion into the pan and sauté until translucent. Place cod steaks in the pan and add tomatoes. Cook for a few minutes, then add capers, olives, and salt and pepper to taste. Cover and cook for 5 minutes. Spoon the sauce over the steaks and sprinkle each one with 1 tablespoon parsley.

BACCALÀ ALLA ANDREAS
Salt Codfish with Vegetables

TIME: 25 MINUTES, EXCLUDING TIME FOR SOAKING COD
SERVINGS: 4
CALORIES: 240 PER SERVING

    1   pound salt codfish
    ½   pound fresh plum tomatoes
    4   white onions, about 1 ounce each
    2   tablespoons olive oil
    2   garlic cloves, peeled
    ¼   cup chopped fresh Italian parsley
    3   tablespoons Spanish capers
    6   small black olives, pitted and chopped

Soak codfish in fresh water to cover for at least 8 hours; if possible, change the water once. Drain cod, rinse, and pat dry. Cut into serving portions. Wash tomatoes, remove hard portion near stem, and chop; there should be 1 cup. Peel and chop onions; there should be ⅓ cup. Heat oil in a large skillet and push garlic through a press into the oil. Add the onions and half of the parsley. Sauté for a few minutes, until onions are translucent. Add cod pieces and brown on both sides. Add tomatoes, capers, olives and remaining parsley. Cover the skillet and cook over medium heat for 15 minutes, or until cod is done to your taste.

BAKED HALIBUT FRANCESCO

TIME: 20 MINUTES
SERVINGS: 10
CALORIES: 250 PER SERVING

    4   pounds fresh halibut steaks, 10 steaks
    1   tablespoon vegetable oil
    1   onion, 2 ounces, peeled
    2   celery ribs
    2   cups dry red wine
    2   whole cloves
    2   pounds fresh tomatoes, chopped
        salt and pepper
    ½   cup chopped fresh Italian parsley

Rinse halibut steaks and pat dry. Use a few drops of the oil to coat a baking dish, and arrange the steaks in it in a single layer. Pour the rest of the oil into a skillet and chop onion and celery into the pan. Sauté until onion is translucent. Add red wine and whole cloves, and cook for a few minutes. Add chopped tomatoes and cook for 6 minutes. Season with salt and pepper to taste, and pour over the halibut steaks. Cover, and bake in a preheated 450°F. oven for 10 minutes, or until fish is just cooked. Sprinkle with parsley and serve.

VARIATIONS: Omit tomatoes for halibut in red-wine sauce.

Place each steak in a layer of heavy-duty foil, spoon some sauce over it, and fold foil to make a secure package. Bake for 10 minutes, or until fish is just cooked.

Instead of wine and tomato sauce, use a sauce of lemon and herbs.

SOLE AND FLOUNDER

Most of the fishes labeled "sole" in American markets are actually flounders. True soles of marketable size are found in European waters, and any fish correctly labeled "Dover sole" in our markets has been imported, probably in a frozen state. However, our flounders, while somewhat thinner through the body, have similar texture and flavor, and can be prepared by the same methods as those used for sole. If you find a recipe calling for sole and cannot find this fish in your market, buy flounder. If you can't find flounder, buy something labeled sole because it will probably be a flounder.

Very small flounder fillets, called "baby flounder," may weigh as little as 2 ounces, but these are more commonly sold to restaurants. The weight of a flounder fillet will range from 3 to 5 ounces, with an average about 4 ounces. These are usually completely boneless, but a few tiny bones may remain at the edges. With a fingertip gently pat along the edges to feel the bone tips, and carefully pull them out.

SOLE LIMONE

TIME: 20 MINUTES
SERVINGS: 4
CALORIES: 140 PER SERVING

4 fillets of sole, 4 ounces each
½ teaspoon vegetable oil
  salt and pepper
3 lemons
½ cup dry white wine
1 teaspoon minced fresh dill
  parsley sprigs

Rinse fillets and pat dry. Coat a baking dish with the oil, and arrange the fillets flat in it. Sprinkle each with a pinch of salt and a dash of pepper. Extract juice from 2 lemons, and cut the third into very thin half slices. Arrange the slices on the fillets, and pour the wine and lemon juice over. Bake in a preheated 400°F. oven for 8 to 10 minutes. Sprinkle with dill and garnish with parsley sprigs, and serve at once.

SOLE WITH CLAM SAUCE

TIME: 25 MINUTES, EXCLUDING TIME TO SHUCK CLAMS
SERVINGS: 4
CALORIES: 205 PER SERVING

1 tablespoon vegetable oil
½ garlic clove, peeled
1 onion, 2 ounces, chopped
½ cup dry white wine
  juice of 1 lemon
1 cup minced fresh clams with juice
½ teaspoon minced fresh tarragon
  dash of white pepper
4 fillets of sole, 4 ounces each
3 tablespoons chopped fresh Italian parsley

Use a few drops of the oil to coat a baking dish. Pour the rest into a skillet and heat. Push garlic through a press into the oil and add the onion; sauté until onion is translucent. Add wine, lemon juice and clams with their natural juice; cook for 2 minutes. Add tarragon and pepper; cook for 4 minutes longer. Rinse fillets, pat dry, and arrange flat in the oiled baking pan. Pour the sauce over the fish, and top with the parsley. Bake in a preheated 400°F. oven for 15 minutes.

VARIATIONS: Lacking good fresh clams, use 7½ ounces canned minced clams, but add these just before the sauce is finished—only long enough to be heated —as these are already cooked.

For a festive version of this, add ½ pound fresh mushrooms. Trim, wash, and dry them, and cut into thin slices or chop them. Sauté with the garlic and onion.

SOLE GRITTI PALACE

TIME: 15 MINUTES
SERVINGS: 4
CALORIES: 350 PER SERVING

> 4 *fillets of sole, 4 ounces each*
> 3 *white onions, 3 ounces each*
> 3 *tablespoons olive oil*
> ½ *cup white raisins*
> 1 *cup dry white wine*
> ¼ *cup dry Marsala wine*
> 2 *tablespoons white vinegar*
> *parsley sprigs*
> *lemon slices*

Rinse fillets and pat dry. Peel onions and cut from top to bottom into thin slices. Heat oil in a large skillet and sauté fish for 2 minutes. Turn fillets over and add onion slices, raisins, both wines and the vinegar, and cook for 10 minutes. Serve with parsley sprigs and lemon slices. This is also good served cold.

VARIATION: Mix oil, wines, onion slices and raisins and marinate the fish in the mixture for 1 to 2 hours before cooking for a stronger-flavored sauce.

SOLE SUPREMA

TIME: 20 TO 25 MINUTES
SERVINGS: 4
CALORIES: 220 PER SERVING

4 *fillets of sole, 4 ounces each*
2 *tablespoons vegetable oil*
2 *pounds fresh tomatoes*
1 *onion, 1 ounce, chopped*
6 *fresh mushrooms, sliced*
2 *tablespoons chopped fresh Italian parsley*
2 *tablespoons chopped fresh basil*
  pepper
5 *pitted black olives, chopped*
4 *parsley sprigs*

Rinse fillets and pat dry. Use a few drops of the oil to coat a baking dish, and arrange the fillets flat in it. Wash and peel tomatoes and chop. Let them drain so the sauce is not watery; the drained juices can be used for soup. Pour the rest of the oil into a skillet and heat. Add onion and mushrooms and sauté until onion is translucent. Add drained tomatoes, chopped parsley and basil, and a dash of pepper. Cook, stirring occasionally, for 6 minutes. Pour the mixture over the sole and top with the olives. Bake in a preheated 400°F. oven for 10 to 12 minutes. Garnish with parsley and serve.

VARIATION: If you lack good ripe tomatoes, use a 2-pound can of peeled whole tomatoes. Let them drain, and break them up with a wooden spoon before adding to the skillet.

SOLE ALLA HENRI

TIME: 20 MINUTES
SERVINGS: 4
CALORIES: 195 PER SERVING

4 *fillets of sole, 4 ounces each*
½ *pound fresh plum tomatoes*
2 *tablespoons olive oil*
3 *large shallots, peeled*
1 *teaspoon crushed red pepper*
3 *tablespoons chopped fresh Italian parsley*
2 *tablespoons chopped fresh basil*
½ *teaspoon crumbled dried orégano*
10 *pitted ripe olives, sliced*
2 *tablespoons capers*

Rinse fillets and pat dry. Wash tomatoes, remove hard portion near stem, and chop tomatoes; there should be 1 cup. Pour oil into a large skillet and chop shallots into the oil. Add crushed pepper and sauté until shallots are translucent. Add tomatoes and herbs and cook for 5 minutes. Gently place sole fillets in the pan and add olives and capers. Cover the pan and poach over low heat for 10 minutes.

VARIATIONS: Add garlic, put through a press, and sliced fresh mushrooms with the shallots.
Use dry white wine instead of tomatoes.

SOLE STUFFED WITH SPINACH

TIME: 15 TO 20 MINUTES
SERVINGS: 4 (2 SMALL ROLLS)
CALORIES: 155 PER SERVING

4 fillets of sole or flounder, 4 ounces each
   salt and pepper
1 cup chopped cooked fresh spinach
½ cup skim-milk cottage or ricotta cheese
½ teaspoon grated nutmeg
¼ cup chopped fresh Italian parsley
½ cup dry white wine
   juice of ½ lemon

Spread the fillets out flat, and separate each one at the center seam, giving 2 narrow fillets from each one. Sprinkle lightly with salt and pepper. Mix spinach, cheese and nutmeg together in a small bowl. Season to your taste with salt and pepper. Place 1 tablespoon of spinach mixture in the center of each strip of fish. Fold one end of the fillet over the filling, then the other end over that, making a three-fold package. Fasten each one with a wooden food pick or a small skewer. Place in a baking dish just large enough to hold the rolls in a single layer. Sprinkle the parsley over the rolls. Mix wine and lemon juice, and spoon over the rolls, dividing it evenly. Bake in a preheated 350°F. oven for 10 minutes, or until done to your taste. Spoon the wine and lemon juice from the pan over the servings for a sauce.

VARIATIONS: Instead of sole or flounder, this dish can be made with fillets of red snapper or striped bass. If the snapper or bass is a large fish, you may wish to cut the fillets into halves crosswise as well as along the center seam to get pieces of appropriate size.

Instead of spinach-cheese filling, try a ricotta filling flavored with chopped fresh dill. Other possibilities are puréed vegetables other than spinach, or chopped mushrooms.

SAUCE VARIATIONS: Instead of the white wine and lemon juice, use any of the following:
> white wine mixed with prepared Dijon mustard and minced fresh dill;
> white wine mixed with curry powder and drained capers;
> Ricotta Sauce (p. 236);
> Tomato Sauce (p. 245).

SAUTÉED FLOUNDER WITH DILL AND SHALLOTS

TIME: 7 MINUTES
SERVINGS: 4
CALORIES: 135 PER SERVING

> 4 flounder fillets, 4 ounces each
> 2 tablespoons vegetable oil
> 6 shallots, peeled
> ¼ cup chopped fresh dill
>   salt and pepper

Rinse fillets and pat dry. These will be turned over once in cooking. If you have a pancake turner wide enough to slide under the whole fillet, fine. If not, it is better to divide fillets lengthwise along the natural center division, as the narrow half-fillet is easier to turn. Heat the oil in a large skillet, chop shallots into it, and sauté them until translucent. Add dill and heat for 1 minute. Gently place fillets in the pan on top of dill and sauté for 2 minutes. Carefully but quickly turn over and cook for 1 minute longer. During this minute sprinkle each fillet with a tiny pinch of salt and a grind of pepper; do not overdo either salt or pepper. Serve fillets at once; flounder fillets are so thin they will be fully cooked. Scoop out some of the dill and shallots to serve with each fillet; most of the oil should be left in the pan.

VARIATIONS: Add garlic; use parsley instead of dill; sprinkle lemon juice over each fillet when serving. Other fillets can be prepared this way, but if they are thicker they will need to cook a little longer.

STRIPED BASS WITH MARINARA SAUCE

TIME: 25 MINUTES
SERVINGS: 6
CALORIES: 205 PER SERVING

1   *whole striped bass, about 4 pounds*
2   *tablespoons vegetable oil*
1   *onion, 2 ounces, chopped*
2   *tablespoons chopped fresh Italian parsley*
½   *teaspoon Italian seasoning*
½   *pound fresh plum tomatoes*
1   *bay leaf*
     salt and pepper

Have fish market scale and dress the fish, and score along both sides from
head to tail. Rinse fish and pat dry. Use a few drops of the oil to coat a baking
dish large enough to hold the bass, and place fish in it. Heat remaining oil
in a skillet and sauté onion, parsley and Italian seasoning until onion is
translucent. Wash tomatoes, remove hard portion near stem, and chop; there
should be 1 cup. Add tomatoes and bay leaf to skillet and cook for 8 minutes.
Add salt and pepper to taste. Pour over the bass and bake in a preheated
400°F. oven for 10 to 15 minutes.

BAKED FISH WITH FENNEL

TIME: 20 MINUTES
SERVINGS: 6
CALORIES: 170 PER SERVING

2   *pounds fillets of halibut, flounder or black sea bass*
1   *tablespoon vegetable oil*
½   *cup dry white wine*
     juice of 1 lemon
     salt and pepper
3   *tablespoons chopped fresh Italian parsley*
¾   *cup chopped fennel leaves (leaves from 2 large bulbs)*

Rinse fish fillets and pat dry. Brush part of the oil on a large baking dish, or
use several dishes if you have a larger amount of fish. Arrange fillets in the
oiled dish, overlapping the pieces slightly if necessary. Pour the wine and

lemon juice over the fish, and sprinkle with a little salt and a tiny dash of pepper. Scatter the green herbs evenly over everything. Cover closely with a sheet of foil, oiled on the side next the fish. Bake in a 400°F. oven for 15 minutes, or less if the fish is done sooner.

VARIATIONS: Instead of parsley and fennel, use chopped olives and a small amount of grated onion.

Instead of herbs, use 2 ounces of anchovies, patted dry to remove excess oil, and chopped or mashed, mixed with 2 large pimientos, chopped. If you use anchovies, add no salt.

Try a mixture of the herbs with any one of the variations.

POACHED FISH ALLA LIVORNESE

TIME: 15 TO 20 MINUTES
SERVINGS: 6
CALORIES: 180 PER SERVING

> 2 *pounds boneless fish fillets (snapper, sole, striped bass, etc.)*
> 1 *pound fresh ripe plum tomatoes, or 2 cups canned peeled plum*
>   *tomatoes*
> 2 *tablespoons vegetable oil*
> 4 *shallots, peeled*
> ¼ *cup dry white wine*
> 3 *tablespoons capers*
> 4 *sprigs of Italian parsley, chopped*
>   *salt and pepper*

Cut fish into 6 portions, rinse, and pat dry. Wash fresh tomatoes, remove hard portion near stem, and chop; there should be 2 cups. (Chop canned tomatoes if that is what you are using.) Heat oil in a large skillet. Mince shallots into the oil and sauté until translucent. Place fish pieces in the pan and add wine and capers. Cook for 2 minutes. Add tomatoes, parsley, and salt and pepper to taste. Cover the pan and poach the fish for 6 to 10 minutes. After 6 minutes, check with a fork. Cook fish only until white and tender; do not overcook. Check the sauce for taste, and add more salt or black pepper if needed. If you poach in a cooking-serving pan, serve the fish in the pan.

VARIATIONS: Add chopped mushrooms, olives, green peppers or zucchini when sautéing the shallots. The dish can be flavored with garlic; mince or push through a press into the oil along with the shallots.

Add 3 clams per serving. Scrub 18 Little Neck clams and carefully open them; leave the clams in the bottom shell and discard top shells. Add clams in their shells to the skillet for the last 2 minutes of poaching.

BAKED TROUT WITH ALMONDS

TIME: 25 MINUTES
SERVINGS: 4
CALORIES: 305 PER SERVING

4 fresh trout, 1 to 1½ pounds each
1 tablespoon vegetable oil
½ cup dry white wine
¼ cup chopped fresh Italian parsley
  salt and pepper
¼ cup slivered blanched almonds
3 lemons, cut into very thin slices

Have fish market scale and dress the trout. Heads can be removed or not as you please. Coat a baking dish with the oil and arrange trout in it in a single layer. Mix wine and parsley, and spoon over the fish. Sprinkle lightly with salt and pepper. Spoon almonds evenly over fish and arrange the lemon slices on top. (Remove any lemon seeds.) Bake in a preheated 400°F. oven for 20 minutes.

TROTE ALLA AL McCLANE
Trout with Vermouth

TIME: 25 MINUTES, BASED ON SHORTEST TIME FOR MARINATING
SERVINGS: 6
CALORIES: 250 PER SERVING

6 whole fresh trout, 10 ounces each
  salt and pepper
2 tablespoons olive oil
3 tablespoons dry vermouth
1 garlic clove, peeled
3 tablespoons chopped fresh Italian parsley
  juice of 2 lemons

Dress the trout, sprinkle them inside with salt and pepper, and arrange in a single layer in a glass or ceramic container. Mix oil and vermouth. Push garlic through a press into the mixture and add parsley. Stir with a fork and pour over the trout. Let trout marinate for at least 10 minutes, but ideally for 1 hour, turning them over or spooning the marinade over them several times. Lift from marinade and arrange in an oiled shallow baking dish. (If the marinating container is suitable for oven use, trout can be baked in it.) Bake in a preheated 375°F. oven for 10 minutes. Serve hot, with some of the lemon juice sprinkled over each little fish.

TROTE INEZ
Trout with Tarragon

TIME: 25 MINUTES, BASED ON SHORTEST TIME FOR MARINATING
SERVINGS: 6
CALORIES: 265 PER TROUT

6 *whole fresh trout, 10 ounces each*
  salt and pepper
6 *fresh tarragon leaves*
2 *tablespoons olive oil*
½ *cup dry white wine*
1 *garlic clove, peeled*
2 *lemons*
6 *tablespoons chopped fresh Italian parsley*

Dress the trout, sprinkle them inside with salt and pepper, and put 1 tarragon leaf in each one. Arrange fish in a single layer in a glass or ceramic container. Mix oil and wine. Push garlic through a press into the mixture, and grate the rind of the lemons into it. Mix with a fork and pour over the trout. Let trout marinate for a least 10 minutes, or for up to 1 hour, turning them over or spooning the marinade over them several times. Lift from marinade and arrange in an oiled shallow baking dish. (If the marinating container is suitable for oven use, trout can be baked in it.) Bake in a preheated 375°F. oven for 10 minutes. While fish bakes, cut off the white inner peel of the lemons and cut the pulp into small cubes; discard any seeds. Serve trout hot; spoon the lemon cubes over and sprinkle each fish with 1 tablespoon parsley.

SEAFOOD WITH WHITE-WINE AND DILL SAUCE

This makes a delicate summer dish. The possibilities are enormous, since it can be made with most species of fish and shellfish, depending on the supplies in your market or your catch. The calories per serving will vary from 150 to 250 according to the kind of seafood you use, and the cooking time will vary in the same fashion, but the average time is 10 minutes.

Prepare White-Wine and Dill Sauce (p. 247). Dress the seafood, according to its type, rinse, and pat dry. Arrange seafood in a single layer in a baking dish and pour the sauce over. Bake uncovered in a preheated 350°F. oven for about 10 minutes, until done to your taste.

For 4 servings prepare 1 pound boneless fish or shelled shellfish.

FISH SOUP ABRUZZO STYLE

TIME: 25 MINUTES
SERVINGS: 6
CALORIES: 195 PER SERVING, EXCLUDING TOAST

> 2 *pounds dressed fresh fish (cod, halibut, sea bass or shellfish), weighed after dressing*
> ½ *pound fresh plum tomatoes*
> 6 *to 8 shallots*
> 3 *tablespoons olive oil*
> 1 *garlic clove, peeled*
> ¼ *cup chopped fresh Italian parsley*
> ⅓ *teaspoon Italian seasoning*
> 1 *cup water*
> 3 *tablespoons white-wine vinegar*
>   *salt and pepper*
> 6 *slices of Italian whole-wheat bread, toasted*

Cut fish into small pieces. Wash tomatoes, remove hard portion near stem, and chop; there should be 1 cup. Peel and chop shallots; there should be ⅓ cup. Heat oil in a 3-quart pot and push garlic through a press into the oil. Add shallots and half of parsley, and sauté until shallots are translucent. Add tomatoes, cook for 2 or 3 minutes, then add Italian seasoning, water and pieces of fish. Cover the pot and cook for 5 minutes. Add vinegar; do not cover the pot, but cook rapidly for a few minutes until liquid is reduced. Add salt and pepper to taste, and stir in remaining parsley. Serve with toasted slices of Italian whole-wheat bread.

VENETIAN FISH STEW

TIME: STOCK—1¼ HOURS; STEW—25 MINUTES
SERVINGS: 4
CALORIES: 300 PER SERVING (BASED ON SEA BASS AND SHRIMPS),
            INCLUDING TOAST

> 2 *pounds assorted fish and shellfish (bass, cod, clams, mussels,*
>   *shrimps, etc.)*
>   *salt*
> 1 *onion, 3 ounces, peeled and sliced*
> 1 *large bay leaf*
> 2 *parsley sprigs with stems*
> 1 *pound fresh plum tomatoes*
> 3 *tablespoons olive oil*
> 2 *garlic cloves, peeled*
> 3 *shallots, peeled*
> 1 *onion, 4 ounces, peeled*
> ¼ *cup chopped fresh Italian parsley*
> ¼ *cup chopped fresh basil*
> ½ *cup dry white wine*
> ⅓ *teaspoon crumbled dried thyme*
> 4 *slices of whole-wheat Italian bread*

FISH STOCK

Dress the fish, saving all heads, bones and trimmings. Discard shells from shellfish. Make fish stock: Put heads and trimmings into a large kettle and cover with 6 cups water. Add ½ tablespoon salt. Toss in onion slices, bay leaf and parsley sprigs. Bring to a boil and simmer for 1 hour. Strain through a coarse sieve, then again through a fine sieve lined with cheesecloth. There should be about 3 cups of strained stock. Set aside.

STEW

While stock is straining, wash tomatoes and cut out hard portion near stem. Chop tomatoes; there should be 2 cups. Cut the boneless dressed fish into 1-inch pieces. Large shrimps can be split. Heat the oil in a deep saucepan and push garlic through a press into the oil. Chop shallots and onion into the pan. Sauté until onion is translucent. Add fish pieces, parsley and basil, and brown fish on both sides. Pour in wine, 3 cups stock and the tomatoes, and add thyme. Simmer for 10 minutes.

    While stew is simmering, toast the bread slices until quite hard, or sauté them in 1 tablespoon olive oil. Serve stew with hard bread slices.

ZUPPA DI PESCHE DEZIAH

TIME: 25 MINUTES
SERVINGS: 6 AS MAIN COURSE; 8 AS SOUP COURSE
CALORIES: 175 PER MAIN-COURSE SERVING; 130 PER SOUP SERVING,
              EXCLUDING TOAST

2 *pounds dressed fresh fish (cod, flounder, Greenland halibut,
  snapper, etc.), weighed after dressing*
6 *cups water*
¼ *cup chopped celery*
4 *shallots, peeled and chopped*
6 *tablespoons chopped fresh Italian parsley*
⅓ *teaspoon Italian seasoning*
1 *bay leaf*
  pinch of cayenne pepper
2 *tablespoons olive oil*
2 *garlic cloves, peeled*
3 *tablespoons dry white wine*
2 *tablespoons tomato paste*
6 *or more slices of Italian bread, toasted hard*

Cut the fish into individual portions for main course, or into smaller chunks
for soup course. Use a 3-quart pot. Pour in the 6 cups of water and add celery,
shallots, 4 tablespoons of the parsley, Italian seasoning, bay leaf and cayenne.
Start adding the fish, beginning with tougher species such as Greenland
halibut and snapper. Bring water to a boil and simmer the tougher species
for 5 minutes. Add tender species and cook for 8 to 10 minutes longer, until
all the kinds of fish are tender. In the meantime make garlic sauce. Pour the
oil into a skillet and push garlic through a press into the oil. Add remaining
2 tablespoons parsley and sauté for a few minutes. Add wine and tomato
paste to garlic and cook until mixed. Turn into the kettle of soup and cook
altogether for 5 minutes. Serve over the hard bread slices in deep soup plates,
dividing the kinds of fish among the plates.

VARIATIONS: Add other kinds of fish; even some tender species not usually
cooked in soups or chowders can be used in this soup, since it is cooked for
such a short time and simmered rather than boiled.

    Shellfish can be used also: shelled clams, mussels, shrimps, squids.
Remember not to overcook these; add them only at the end, with the garlic
sauce.

FISH AND VEGETABLE MISTO

For this one-pot meal a variety of fresh fish and shellfish can be used, either one kind or a mixture; in fact a mixture gives good texture.

TIME: 15 MINUTES
SERVINGS: 4
CALORIES: 215 PER SERVING (BASED ON STRIPED BASS)

> 1 *pound flounder, striped bass or other white-fleshed fish, or 1 pound shelled and deveined shrimps or shelled mussels or scallops*
> 1 *large green pepper*
> 2 *tablespoons oil*
> 1 *garlic clove, peeled*
> 3 *shallots, peeled*
> ¼ *cup chopped celery*
> ¼ *teaspoon crushed red pepper*
> ½ *cup dry white wine*
> ½ *teaspoon Italian seasoning*
> *salt and pepper*
> ¼ *cup chopped fresh Italian parsley*

Dice the fish; if shrimps or scallops are large, they can be split or chopped. Wash and trim green pepper, discard ribs and seeds, and chop pepper. Heat oil in a large pot and push garlic through a press into the oil. Chop shallots into the pan and add celery, green pepper and crushed red pepper. Sauté and stir together for 3 minutes. Add the fish or shellfish, wine and Italian seasoning, and mix. Cook for 5 minutes. Add salt and pepper if needed, and serve sprinkled with parsley.

VARIATIONS: Add chopped mushrooms or chopped zucchini, or substitute these for the celery and green pepper. Other choices are chopped broccoli and diced pimientos.

FRESH CRAB WITH MUSHROOMS

No European crab can compare with the American blue crab, so that's the crab used for this simple preparation. In Italy other crabs would be used. If you can't find fresh crab, don't make this; canned crab is entirely different.

TIME: 10 MINUTES
SERVINGS: 4
CALORIES: 195 PER SERVING

1 *pound cooked fresh blue crab*
¼ *pound small mushrooms*
2 *green Italian peppers (frying peppers)*
4 *shallots*
1 ½ *red pimientos*
2 *tablespoons unsalted butter*
¼ *cup dry white wine*
   salt and white pepper
3 *tablespoons minced fresh Italian parsley*

Unless you have boiled or steamed the crabs and picked them yourself, put the cooked crab into a large strainer and rinse with cold water. Drain well and turn the crab onto a towel. Pick it over carefully to remove any bits of cartilage. Wash and trim mushrooms and pat dry; cut them into quarters. Wash and trim peppers, discard ribs and seeds, and mince. Peel and mince shallots, and chop pimientos. Melt butter in a large skillet and in it sauté shallots and peppers until shallots are translucent. Add mushrooms and pimientos and sauté for 2 minutes. Add crab, gently stir it to mix well with the vegetables, then add wine and simmer for a minute or two, just long enough to heat the crab. Season with salt and white pepper to taste. Sprinkle with parsley and serve at once.

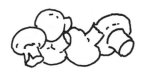

RICCARDO'S LOBSTER FRA DIAVOLO

The lobster found in Italian waters, *aragosta,* is related to the spiny lobster of American southern coastal waters. While live specimens can be purchased in fish markets in Italy, here you will probably need to buy them as frozen "lobster tails." These lobsters have no large claws.

TIME: 25 MINUTES
SERVINGS: 4
CALORIES: 275 PER SERVING

> 8 *frozen lobster tails, 4 ounces each including shell weight*
> 1 *teaspoon salt*
> 1 *tablespoon vinegar*
> 1 *pound fresh plum tomatoes*
> 2 *tablespoons olive oil*
> 2 *garlic cloves, peeled*
> 3 *shallots, peeled*
> ¼ *teaspoon crushed red pepper*
> ¼ *teaspoon crumbled dried orégano*
> ½ *cup white wine*
> ¼ *cup minced fresh Italian parsley*

With kitchen scissors slit both upper and lower shell of frozen tails. Drop them into a large pot with 2 quarts water, the salt and vinegar. Bring to a boil and cook for 5 minutes. Drain tails, rinse in cold water to cool them, then carefully extract meat from shells. Cut each tail into round medallions. Wash and peel tomatoes, remove hard portion near stem, and chop.

Heat oil in a large skillet and push garlic through a press into the oil. Chop shallots into the oil and add red pepper. When shallots are translucent, add lobster medallions and sauté over brisk heat for 1 minute on each side. Remove lobster to a plate and add chopped tomatoes, orégano and wine to the skillet. Cover and simmer for 10 minutes. Return lobster pieces to skillet, heat for 1 minute, and add parsley. Heat for another minute, then serve at once.

VARIATIONS: You can make this more "devilish" by adding more crushed red pepper or cayenne.

MUSSELS IN WHITE WINE

TIME: 20 MINUTES
SERVINGS: 4
CALORIES: 135 PER SERVING OF 12 MUSSELS

> 2 *pounds mussels in shells*
> 1 *onion, 2 ounces*
> 3 *small garlic cloves*
> 2 *celery ribs*
> ½ *bunch of Italian parsley*
> 1 *cup dry white wine*
>   *dash of black pepper*

Scrub mussels with a stiff brush or plastic pot scrubber, and remove beards. Discard any that are open. Put mussels in a large pot or kettle and cover with cold water. Peel onion and garlic; wash celery and parsley; chop all these vegetables. Lift mussels out of the water and let them drain. Empty the pot and rinse out any sand. Return mussels to the empty pot, and add chopped vegetables, wine and a dash of pepper. Cover the pot and bring the liquid to a boil. Let the mussels steam for 5 minutes, or longer if you prefer, until the shells open. For even cooking, stir them once during steaming. Using a skimmer, lift out mussels, letting any juices fall into the pan. Discard any unopened shells. Strain the broth through a fine sieve, and divide it among the soup bowls. Divide the mussels, still in their shells, among the bowls and serve at once, with oyster forks and soup spoons. Be sure to drink the broth.

MUSSELS AND SHRIMPS JUDY

TIME: 20 MINUTES
SERVINGS: 4
CALORIES: 220 PER SERVING

1 pound mussels in shells
1 pound raw shrimps in shells
2 tablespoons unsalted butter
3 shallots, peeled
1 tablespoon brandy
2 tablespoons light cream
½ cup dry Marsala wine
3 tablespoons chopped fresh Italian parsley

Scrub mussels with a stiff brush or plastic pot scrubber, and remove beards. Cover with cold water and let them soak for 5 minutes. Drain, rinse out pot, and return mussels to the pot. Add 1 cup water and steam mussels for 5 minutes, until all shells are open. Discard shells; there should be about 1 cup of mussels. Shell and devein shrimps. Melt butter in a skillet and chop shallots into the pan. Sauté shrimps and shallots for 3 minutes. Add brandy and cream and simmer for a few minutes. Add mussels, then Marsala, and cook for 3 minutes. Sprinkle with parsley, or stir it in. Serve with rice or as a pasta sauce.

MUSSEL AND SHRIMP SALAD

TIME: 15 MINUTES, EXCLUDING TIME FOR CHILLING
SERVINGS: 6
CALORIES: 185 PER SERVING

2 *pounds raw mussels in shells*
2 *pounds raw shrimps in shells*
2 *red bell peppers, trimmed and diced*
¼ *cup diced celery*
3 *shallots, peeled and chopped*
3 *tablespoons chopped fresh Italian parsley*
3 *tablespoons snipped fresh dill*
2 *tablespoons vegetable oil*
   juice of 1 lemon
1 *garlic clove, peeled and crushed*
¼ *teaspoon Italian seasoning*
1 *bunch of watercress*

Scrub mussels with a stiff brush or plastic pot scrubber, and remove beards. Cover with cold water. Shell and devein shrimps, and poach for 5 minutes, until they are pink; do not overcook. Lift mussels out of the water and let them drain. Empty the pot and rinse out any sand. Return mussels to the empty pot, add 2 cups water, and steam mussels for 5 minutes, until all the shells are open. Discard any unopened shells. Cool shrimps and mussels. Mix in a bowl with red peppers, celery, shallots, parsley and dill. In a cup mix oil, lemon juice, garlic and Italian seasoning. Pour over the salad and mix well. Remove all stems from watercress and toss leaves into the salad. Chill.

GAMBERETTI ALLA GIUSEPPE
Shrimps with Tomatoes

TIME: 15 MINUTES
SERVINGS: 4
CALORIES: 145 PER SERVING

1 *pound raw shrimps in shells*
2 *tablespoons unsalted butter*
2 *tablespoons capers*
2 *tablespoons brandy*
½ *cup chopped peeled fresh tomatoes (about 4 plum tomatoes)*
2 *tablespoons tomato paste*

Shell and devein shrimps, and cook in butter for 3 minutes. Add capers and brandy and cook for a few minutes. Add fresh tomatoes and simmer for 5 minutes, then blend in tomato paste and cook for 2 minutes. Serve with rice or pasta.

VARIATION: To make *scampi alla Giuseppe,* use lobsterettes, which you will find frozen in U.S. markets. Defrost lobsterettes in the refrigerator overnight, and shell before using.

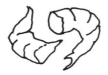

GAMBERETTI LICIA
Shrimps in Garlic-Wine Sauce

This can also be served as a first course; it will make 6 to 8 servings.

TIME: 15 MINUTES
SERVINGS: 4
CALORIES: 250 PER SERVING

    2 *pounds raw shrimps in shells*
    3 *tablespoons olive oil*
    2 *garlic cloves, peeled*
    ½ *cup chopped fresh Italian parsley*
    ⅓ *teaspoon Italian seasoning*
    ¼ *teaspoon cayenne pepper*
    ½ *cup dry white wine*
       salt and pepper

Shell shrimps, devein if necessary, rinse, and roll in paper towels to dry. Heat the oil in a large skillet and push garlic through a press into the oil. Add shrimps and parsley and sauté for a few minutes. Sprinkle in Italian seasoning and cayenne, then pour in the wine; stir. Cook for 3 minutes, or until the wine evaporates. Shrimps will be bright pink. Season with salt and pepper to taste. Serve with rice or boiled potatoes and a green vegetable.

GAMBERETTI ALLA ENNIO
Shrimps in Garlic Sauce

TIME: 20 MINUTES
SERVINGS: 4
CALORIES: 238 PER SERVING

> 2 pounds raw jumbo shrimps in shells
> 3 tablespoons vegetable oil
> 3 garlic cloves, peeled
> 2 shallots, peeled
> ¼ cup dry Marsala wine
>   juice of 1 lemon
> ¼ cup chopped fresh Italian parsley
> 1 cup tomato sauce

Shell and devein shrimps. Rinse and pat dry. Heat oil in a skillet. Push garlic through a press into the oil, and mince the shallots into the oil as well. Sauté for a minute or two. Add shrimps and toss in the oil. Add wine, lemon juice and parsley, and cook for a few minutes longer. Add tomato sauce and cook for 5 minutes. Serve hot over rice.

SHRIMPS IN TOMATO-HERB SAUCE

This recipe can be used as a first course or main dish.

TIME: 15 MINUTES
SERVINGS: 4
CALORIES: 220 PER SERVING

> 2 pounds raw medium-size shrimps in shells
> 2 tablespoons vegetable oil
> 6 to 8 fresh plum tomatoes, peeled, chopped and drained (1 cup chopped)
> ¼ cup chopped fresh Italian parsley
> 1 tablespoon Italian seasoning
> ½ tablespoon chopped fresh basil
> ½ small garlic clove, crushed
>   salt and pepper

Rinse raw shrimps, peel, and devein. Pour the oil into a large frying pan, and add chopped tomatoes, parsley, Italian seasoning, basil and garlic. Cook over medium heat for 2 minutes. Season with salt and pepper to taste. Add shrimps and cook for 6 to 8 minutes, until shrimps are pink and tender. Do not overcook. Stir often to mix shrimps with sauce.

VARIATIONS: Instead of shrimps, use *scampi,* which you may find in your market labeled "lobsterettes," "Danish lobster tails," or "prawns." (They are actually lobsterettes.)

Instead of tomatoes, use 1 cup sautéed chopped mushrooms, or green peppers, or onions, or zucchini, or a mixture of two or more of the vegetables.

Instead of tomatoes, use ½ cup dry red wine.

CALAMARI ALLA LUCIO
Squid in Tomato Sauce

TIME: 20 MINUTES
SERVINGS: 4
CALORIES: 200 PER SERVING

> 1 ½ *pounds small squids*
> ½ *pound fresh plum tomatoes*
> 1 *onion, 4 ounces*
> ¼ *cup blanched almonds*
> 1 *tablespoon vegetable oil*
> 1 *garlic clove, peeled*
> ¼ *cup chopped fresh Italian parsley*
> 1 *teaspoon grated lemon rind*
> ¼ *teaspoon crumbled dried rosemary*
>   *salt and white pepper*

Buy the smallest squids available, for they will be most tender and most quickly cooked. Dress them: remove mantle, head, and rudimentary shell (like a piece of transparent plastic). With the fingers peel off the purple skin (it is edible, but it discolors the dish). Cut squid into small strips. Wash tomatoes, remove hard portion near stem, and chop; there should be 1 cup. Peel and mince onion. Grind or chop almonds; they should be reduced to very small crumbs. Heat oil in a skillet and push garlic through a press into the oil. Add onion and half of the parsley and sauté until onion is translucent. Add tomatoes, lemon rind and rosemary, and simmer for 8 minutes. Add squid strips and ground almonds and cook over low heat for about 3 minutes. Squid is edible raw; if it is overcooked, it develops a rubbery texture. Taste a piece and stop cooking the minute it is done to suit. Season with salt and white pepper to taste, and stir in the rest of the parsley. Serve at once.

CHICKEN AND GAME

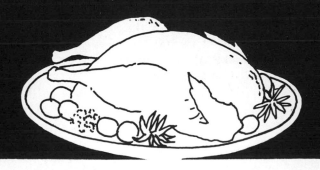

There is an old European saying: "The kitchen that has a chicken in the pot is a household that is warm and friendly and has a good cook."

The meat of the chicken provides a complete protein and some valuable vitamins and as a plus is low in calories. At present chicken is also economical. Its natural affinity for wines, herbs and spices makes it a perfect food for the imaginative cook. The recipes in this chapter will be useful for everyday cooking routines as well as for entertaining. Also there are variations that can be developed to your taste based on ingredients which you already have in your cupboard.

All kinds of chickens and related birds, even the tiny Rock Cornish hens, are available fresh. Don't be tempted to purchase them frozen. If you have been cooking and eating only frozen birds for some time, you may be surprised at the flavor and juiciness of fresh poultry. When a frozen bird is defrosted there is considerable loss of juice, and with that juice goes flavor and vitamins. A fresh chicken can be stored in your refrigerator for 3 days without spoiling, and chicken is always to be found in markets. The apparent convenience of frozen storage turns out not to be so convenient when one adds the time needed for defrosting.

The chickens that we buy today in the United States have been bred to be very tender. Also they are marketed when very young, some as young as 6 to 8 weeks. Because they are so young and the flesh so delicate, cooking time is very important. As with fish and veal, the second the meat goes past the raw-pink stage, you must spoon in whatever sauces or juices are required for the dish, and continue to cook only until just done. Chicken becomes tough and tasteless if overcooked. Use low to medium heat. With a sharp knife slash the cooked portion as soon as it is turned over in the pan; in this way you can check the color of the meat near the center.

While other flavorings may be added early on, seasoning with salt should come later. The salt shaker seems an inevitable accompaniment to our cooking, but hold back! The flesh of chickens has some natural salt, but it has a special flavor of its own that you may not wish to alter by salting at all. If you do use salt, add it at the end. Salt toughens the protein of chicken and extracts juices when added during cooking.

An American specialty is the broiler-fryer, a tender young bird of 2½ to 3 pounds. It is this size of bird that is used in these recipes, and the chicken breasts used come from birds of that size. You will notice that most of the recipes call for "skinless" pieces; the skin has a fatty layer and it is best to remove it for low-caiorie cooking.

In addition to chicken dishes you will find in this chapter recipes for quail and rabbit, both popular in Italy.

POLLO ALLA FIORENTINA
Chicken with Mushrooms and White Wine

TIME: 25 MINUTES
SERVINGS: 8
CALORIES: 225 PER SERVING

1 cup dried black mushrooms (about 2 ounces)
2 frying chickens, 2½ pounds each
1 white onion, 4 ounces
½ pound fresh plum tomatoes
1 teaspoon olive oil
3 tablespoons chopped lean bacon
salt and pepper
¾ cup dry white wine
⅓ cup chopped fresh Italian parsley
3 tablespoons chopped fresh basil

Soak mushrooms in hot water while preparing other ingredients. Cut chickens into pieces; divide half-breasts into 2 portions; save backs and necks for stock. Remove all skin. Peel and chop the onion. Wash tomatoes and cut out hard portion near stem. Chop tomatoes; there should be about 1 cup. Heat oil and bacon bits in a large skillet until bacon begins to cook. Add chopped onion and sauté until onion is translucent. Brown chicken pieces on all sides in the same pan, then sprinkle lightly with salt and pepper. Add wine, parsley, basil and tomatoes. Drain mushrooms, remove stems (save for something else), and cut caps with scissors into thin slivers. Add mushrooms to the mixture, cover the skillet, and cook for 10 minutes, or until chicken is done to your taste.

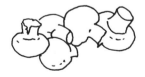

CHICKEN IN GARLIC SAUCE

TIME: 15 TO 20 MINUTES
SERVINGS: 4
CALORIES: 230 PER SERVING

4 *half-breasts of chicken, boneless and skinless, 5 ounces each*
2 *tablespoons olive oil*
4 *garlic cloves, peeled*
½ *cup chicken stock*
½ *cup dry white wine*
  salt and pepper
¼ *cup chopped fresh Italian parsley*

Rinse chicken pieces and pat dry. Heat oil in a large skillet, and push garlic through a press into the oil. Add chicken and sauté for 2 minutes on each side. Slash each piece so you can check the color. Add stock and wine and bring to a boil. Reduce heat, cover the pan, and cook for 5 minutes, or until the color of the inside shows the chicken is done. Do not overcook. Add salt and pepper to taste and sprinkle with parsley.

VARIATION: Add 1 cup sliced fresh mushrooms, or use ½ cup (about 1 ounce) dried black mushrooms. Prepare them as described in the recipe for Mushroom Risotto (p. 93).

CHICKEN LIMONE

TIME: 12 TO 15 MINUTES
SERVINGS: 4
CALORIES: 165 PER SERVING

1 *pound boneless and skinless white meat of chicken*
1 *tablespoon unsalted butter*
  salt and white pepper
½ *cup dry white wine*
4 *lemons*

Rinse chicken and pat dry. Cut into bite-size pieces. Melt the butter in a skillet and add chicken pieces. Sauté for 2 or 3 minutes, turning each piece once. Sprinkle lightly with salt and pepper, then add wine and the juice of 2 lemons. Slice remaining lemons into very thin slices, discard any seeds, and add slices to chicken. Cover the pan and simmer for 5 minutes. Serve hot or cold.

CHICKEN MARSALA

TIME: 10 TO 12 MINUTES
SERVINGS: 4
CALORIES: 220 PER SERVING

4 half-breasts of chicken, boneless and skinless, 5 ounces each
1 tablespoon unsalted butter
4 shallots, peeled
½ cup dry Marsala wine
  salt and pepper

Rinse chicken and pat dry. Heat butter in a skillet and mince the shallots into the pan. Add chicken and sauté on one side. Turn over; slash across the center to check the color. Add wine, turn the pieces in the wine, and cook for 5 minutes, until the inside of the chicken is white. Add salt and pepper to taste.

CHICKEN PARMA

TIME: 15 TO 20 MINUTES
SERVINGS: 8
CALORIES: 175 PER SERVING

8 small chicken parts, about 3 pounds altogether
2 tablespoons vegetable oil
1 onion, 4 ounces, peeled and chopped
½ cup chopped fresh mushrooms
1 cup dry white wine
¼ cup chopped fresh Italian parsley
1 teaspoon Italian seasoning
½ teaspoon snipped fresh tarragon
6 tablespoons tomato paste
6 red Italian olives, pitted and sliced

Remove skin from chicken pieces, rinse pieces, and pat dry. Heat oil in a large skillet and brown chicken pieces on all sides. Add onion and mushrooms and sauté until onion is translucent. Add wine, half of parsley, the Italian seasoning and tarragon; simmer for 1 minute. Add tomato paste and olives, cover, and simmer for about 5 minutes, until chicken is cooked. If you have both white meat and dark meat, the dark may need an extra minute for tenderness, but be sure not to overcook the white meat pieces. Sprinkle with remaining parsley. Serve hot with noodles or rice.

VARIATION: Use dried mushrooms instead of fresh. For method, see Mushroom Risotto (p. 93).

POLLO ALL'ARRABBIATA
Chicken with Hot Pepper Sauce

TIME: 25 MINUTES
SERVINGS: 8
CALORIES: 260 PER SERVING

> 2 *frying chickens, 2½ pounds each*
> 1 *dried tiny chili pepper*
> ½ *pound fresh plum tomatoes*
> 3 *tablespoons vegetable oil*
> *salt and pepper*
> 1½ *cups dry white wine*
> ⅓ *cup chopped fresh Italian parsley*

Cut chickens into pieces; divide half-breasts into 2 portions; save backs and necks for stock. Remove all skin. With plastic or rubber gloves, slit the chili pepper and rinse away all seeds; cut out stem and any ribs. Still wearing gloves, chop the pepper to fine bits. Wash tomatoes and cut out hard portion near stem. Chop tomatoes; there should be about 1 cup; let them drain. Heat oil in a large skillet and sauté chicken pieces until golden brown on all sides. Season the pieces with salt and pepper after they are browned. Pour in the wine and simmer for a few minutes. Add tomatoes, chopped chili pepper and parsley. Cover the pot, reduce heat, and cook for 10 minutes, or until chicken is done to your taste.

CHICKEN SARNA
Chicken with Mustard and Capers

TIME: 10 MINUTES
SERVINGS: 4
CALORIES: 210 PER SERVING

4 half-breasts of chicken, 5 ounces each, boneless and skinless
6 shallots
3 sprigs of Italian parsley
½ pound fresh mushrooms
½ cup dry white wine
½ teaspoon minced fresh tarragon
¼ cup unsalted capers
3 tablespoons prepared Dijon mustard
*   black pepper*

Wipe chicken breasts with a cloth dipped into cold water, and pat dry. Flatten slightly with the flat side of a cleaver. Peel shallots. Wash and dry parsley and cut off stems. Wash mushrooms and trim off the bottom of stems.

Pour ¼ cup of the wine into a heavy frying pan, and place over medium to low heat. Chop the shallots into the wine, and slice mushrooms into the pan also. Stir with a wooden spoon. Snip parsley into the pan and add tarragon and capers. Slash chicken breasts across top and bottom and add to pan. Cook for 2 minutes. Mix remaining wine, the mustard, and black pepper to taste and pour over chicken. Turn the chicken and check the inside, where the slashes are, to help with timing. Cook just past the pink stage to keep chicken tender, about 8 minutes altogether. If the pan gets dry, add a little more white wine and keep turning the chicken until done to your taste.

Serve onto plates, with the pan sauce poured on top, and sprinkle with a little freshly ground pepper. Accompany with rice and a green vegetable.

VARIATIONS: Add more mustard or wine or capers to your taste. Keep tasting the sauce as you cook to be sure the taste is just right.

Omit capers or mushrooms.

Instead of tarragon, use 3 sprigs of fresh dill, snipped.

Serve cold, garnished with lots of fresh dill.

CHICKEN AND EGGPLANT MISTO

TIME: 20 TO 25 MINUTES
SERVINGS: 6
CALORIES: 160 PER SERVING

> 3 eggplants, about 12 ounces each
> salt
> ½ cup dry red wine
> 2 half-breasts of chicken, boneless and skinless, 5 ounces each
> 2 tablespoons vegetable oil
> 1 tablespoon olive oil
> 4 shallots, peeled
> 2 garlic cloves, peeled
> ¼ cup chopped fresh Italian parsley
> ¼ teaspoon Italian seasoning
> 4 black Italian olives, pitted and chopped
> pepper

Wash eggplants and remove stem and leaves but do not peel. Cut eggplants into cubes and drop cubes into a large pan of cold water with ¼ cup salt. Soak for a few minutes, then drain, rinse thoroughly, and drain again. Place in a single layer in a shallow baking dish and slide under the broiler for 5 minutes. Sprinkle cubes with a few drops of the red wine during the broiling. Set the baking dish of eggplant cubes aside.

While eggplant is soaking and broiling, prepare the chicken. Dice the boneless meat. Heat all the oil in a large skillet. Chop shallots into the oil and push the garlic through a press into the pan. Add half of the parsley and the chicken dice, and sauté for a few minutes, turning the pieces over during cooking. Add the rest of the wine, the eggplant cubes, Italian seasoning and olives. Cook for 5 minutes, turning to mix everything well. Season with salt and pepper to taste. Add remaining parsley and serve at once.

VARIATIONS: Use tomato sauce instead of wine.

Use zucchini instead of eggplant, or a mixture of eggplant and zucchini.

ROBERTO'S CHICKEN IN VINEGAR SAUCE

TIME: 20 MINUTES, EXCLUDING TIME FOR CHILLING
SERVINGS: 4
CALORIES: 260 PER SERVING

1 *frying chicken, 2½ pounds*
1 *green pepper*
3 *pimientos, drained*
2 *tablespoons olive oil*
4 *garlic cloves, peeled*
½ *cup chopped white onions*
¼ *cup red-wine vinegar*
⅓ *cup chopped fresh Italian parsley*
3 *tablespoons drained capers*
2 *whole cloves*
   salt and pepper
4 *lemon wedges*

Cut the chicken into 8 pieces (or have the butcher do this), rinse, and pat dry. (Save back, neck and wing tips for stock.) Wash and trim green pepper, discard ribs and seeds, and cut into thin strips. Dice the pimientos. Heat the oil in a large skillet, and push garlic through a press into the oil. Add chopped onions and green pepper strips. Sauté until onions are translucent. Add chicken pieces and brown on both sides. Add vinegar, parsley, capers, cloves and diced pimientos; cook for 5 minutes. Add salt and pepper to taste, cover, and cook for 5 minutes longer. Uncover and let chicken and sauce cool. Serve cold, with lemon wedges.

CHICKEN AND BEEF SYLVESTER, JR.

TIME: 20 TO 25 MINUTES
SERVINGS: 8
CALORIES: 190 PER SERVING

8 *small chicken parts, all white meat or a mixture of white and*
   dark meat, about 3 pounds altogether
1 *onion, 3 ounces*
1 *large green pepper*
2 *tablespoons vegetable oil*
½ *pound lean beefsteak, ground*
½ *cup dry red wine*
½ *teaspoon crumbled dried orégano*
¼ *teaspoon cayenne pepper*
   salt and black pepper

Discard skin and bones from chicken, and cut the meat into bite-size pieces. Peel and chop onion. Wash and trim green pepper, discard rib and seeds, and chop or sliver the pepper. Heat oil in a large skillet and brown chicken pieces on all sides. With a skimmer lift them out of the oil to a plate. Drop onion and pepper pieces into the skillet and sauté until onion is translucent. Add ground steak and toss in the oil until it is no longer red. Return the chicken to the pan and add wine, orégano and cayenne. Stir to mix, and cook for 2 minutes, or until chicken and beef are done to suit you. Season with salt and black pepper to taste. Serve with rice and a salad.

VARIATIONS: Add chopped or sliced mushrooms with the onion and green pepper, or sliced olives or artichokes with the wine. Use tomato sauce instead of red wine.

ITALIAN CHICKEN STEW

TIME: 25 MINUTES
SERVINGS: 6
CALORIES: 250 PER SERVING

        3 pounds chicken pieces
        ½ pound fresh plum tomatoes
        2 green peppers
        2 red bell peppers
        ½ pound fresh mushrooms
        6 to 8 shallots
        2 tablespoons olive oil
        2 garlic cloves, peeled
        ½ cup chopped celery
        ⅓ teaspoon Italian seasoning
        ⅓ teaspoon crushed red pepper (optional)
            salt and pepper
        ½ cup dry red wine
        ⅓ cup chopped fresh Italian parsley

Remove bones and skin from chicken pieces and cut the meat into 1-inch pieces. Wash tomatoes, remove hard portion near stem, and chop; there should be 1 cup. Wash and trim green and red bell peppers, discard ribs and seeds, and chop peppers. Wash mushrooms and roll in a towel to dry. Remove stems (save for another recipe), and chop the caps. Peel and chop shallots;

there should be ⅓ cup. Heat oil in a large skillet, and push garlic through a press into the oil. Add shallots, celery and green and red bell peppers, and sauté until shallots are translucent and peppers are softened. Add chopped mushrooms, Italian seasoning and crushed red pepper (if you wish), and cook for 2 minutes. Add chicken pieces and sauté them, turning to brown all sides, for 2 or 3 minutes longer. Season chicken pieces with salt and pepper to taste. Add wine, tomatoes and parsley, and cook for 5 minutes, until chicken is done to your taste and the vegetables are tender and well combined. Serve with *risotto.*

VARIATIONS: Use zucchini instead of peppers. Add olives. Use red wine but omit tomatoes. Add chopped cooked artichoke bottoms.

BREAST OF CAPON IN OYSTER SAUCE ALLA ALITALIA

TIME: 20 MINUTES
SERVINGS: 4
CALORIES: 375 PER SERVING

  1 *whole capon breast, about 2½ pounds*
 12 *shucked fresh oysters, with natural juices*
  1 *tablespoon unsalted butter*
  1 *tablespoon vegetable oil*
  ¼ *cup chopped shallots*
  5 *tablespoons chopped fresh Italian parsley*
  ½ *cup dry white wine*
     salt and pepper

Split the capon breast, remove skin and bones, and divide each half into 2 portions. To make 4 even portions, add part of the larger fillet of each half to the smaller fillet; the natural protein will keep these separate pieces together in cooking. Each portion should weigh about 5 ounces. Rinse the oysters and strain the juices through a cloth-lined sieve to remove any bits of shell. Reserve the juices, and chop the oysters. Heat butter and oil in a large skillet and add shallots. When shallots are translucent, add 3 table-spoons of the parsley. Sauté for 1 minute, then add capon pieces and sauté for about 3 minutes on each side. Slash across the center of breast pieces to check on degree of pinkness. Add oysters and wine and cook for a few minutes, only long enough to heat oysters and blend flavors. If the pan begins to dry, add a little of the reserved oyster juices. When capon is done to your taste and oysters are hot, add remaining parsley and season with salt and pepper to taste. Serve with rice.

CHICKEN LIVERS

Of all edible livers, these are the lowest in calories, less than 190 calories for ¼ pound simmered, which is a typical serving. There is no waste. They contain valuable protein but little fat. Chicken livers can be prepared in many interesting sauces—brown sauce made with onions, red-wine sauce (which the Italians prefer), white-wine sauce, mushroom sauce, cream sauce, tomato sauce. Livers can also be mixed with vegetables, pasta and *risotto*. Venice is the region famous for great dishes prepared with chicken livers *(fegato)*.

Buy only fresh chicken livers from your butcher, never frozen livers. If you find them only in plastic containers in your supermarket, buy only those that look fresh or are dated. Rinse them thoroughly in cold water. If you are simmering the livers, use just enough water to cover them, and cook gently until no longer pink; do not let them become dry or hard.

Chicken livers can be used for cocktail food—as a pâté or spread for wheat crackers or vegetables; for a first course—prepared with mushrooms or used to stuff vegetables; for a pasta sauce—see Pasta alla Toscana; for a main dish—in red-wine sauce or any of the other possibilities. From an economic standpoint they are a fantastic bargain.

CHICKEN LIVERS IN RED-WINE SAUCE ALLA CARLO

TIME: 15 MINUTES
SERVINGS: 4
CALORIES: 315 PER SERVING

1 pound fresh chicken livers
   salt
1 slice of bacon
1 yellow onion, about 2 ounces
2 tablespoons vegetable oil
¼ cup chopped fresh Italian parsley
⅛ teaspoon crushed red pepper
1 cup dry red wine
⅓ teaspoon dried basil

Rinse livers, trim if necessary, and put in a saucepan. Cover with cold water, add a pinch of salt, and bring to a boil. Reduce heat and simmer livers for 3 minutes. Drain livers, and cut each one into 2 or 3 pieces. Cut the bacon into tiny dice, and peel and chop onion. Heat oil in a skillet and add bacon dice, onion, parsley and crushed red pepper. Sauté, turning often, until bacon is cooked and onion translucent. Add livers, wine and basil, and simmer until livers are done to your taste and sauce somewhat reduced—a few minutes is enough.

CHICKEN LIVERS WITH MARSALA

TIME: 15 MINUTES
SERVINGS: 4
CALORIES: 260 PER SERVING

  1 *pound fresh chicken livers*
    salt
  6 *fresh mushrooms*
 10 *to 12 shallots*
  1 *tablespoon unsalted butter*
 ¼ *cup chopped fresh Italian parsley*
 ¼ *teaspoon dried basil*
 ½ *cup sweet Marsala wine*

Rinse livers, trim if necessary, and put in a saucepan. Cover with cold water, add a pinch of salt, and bring to a boil. Reduce heat and simmer livers for 4 minutes. Drain livers and cut each one into 2 or 3 pieces. Wash and trim mushrooms, and chop; there should be ½ cup. Peel and mince shallots; there should be ½ cup. Heat butter in a skillet and sauté shallots and mushrooms in it until shallots are translucent and mushrooms lightly browned. Stir often. Add livers, sauté for 1 minute, then add parsley, basil and Marsala. Cook for 3 minutes, or until livers are done to your taste.

VARIATION: Instead of fresh mushrooms, use 6 or more dried black mushrooms. Rinse them, then soak in Marsala for 30 minutes or longer. Use the soaking wine in the sauce.

CHICKEN LIVERS AND PEPPERS

TIME: 15 MINUTES
SERVINGS: 4
CALORIES: 290 PER SERVING

1 *pound fresh chicken livers*
   salt
1 *red bell pepper*
1 *green pepper*
2 *white onions, 1 ½ ounces each*
2 *tablespoons vegetable oil*
¼ *cup chopped fresh Italian parsley*
½ *cup dry red wine*
¼ *teaspoon Italian seasoning*
⅛ *teaspoon crushed red pepper*

Rinse livers, trim if necessary, and put in a saucepan. Cover with cold water, add a pinch of salt, and bring to a boil. Reduce heat and simmer livers for 3 minutes. Drain livers, and cut each one into 2 or 3 pieces. Wash and trim both peppers, discard ribs and seeds, and mince peppers. Peel and chop onions; there should be about ⅓ cup. Heat oil in a skillet and add onions, minced peppers and half of the parsley. Sauté until onions are translucent. Add livers, wine, Italian seasoning, crushed red pepper and remaining parsley. Cover and cook for 3 minutes, or until livers are done to your taste.

CHICKEN LIVERS IN MUSTARD SAUCE
IL BOSCHETTO, BRONX, NEW YORK

TIME: 15 MINUTES
SERVINGS: 4
CALORIES: 260 PER SERVING

1 *pound fresh chicken livers*
   salt
¼ *pound fresh broccoli*
10 *to 12 shallots*
1 *tablespoon unsalted butter*
3 *tablespoons capers*
1 *cup dry white wine*
2 *tablespoons prepared Dijon mustard*
¼ *cup chopped fresh Italian parsley*
1 *tablespoon minced fresh dill*

Rinse chicken livers, trim if necessary, and put in a saucepan. Cover with cold water, add a pinch of salt, and bring to a boil. Reduce heat and simmer livers for 4 minutes. Drain livers and cut each one into 2 or 3 pieces. Wash and trim broccoli, peel stems if necessary, and chop; there should be about ½ cup. Cover broccoli with cold water, add a pinch of salt, bring to a boil, and boil for 4 minutes. Drain and at once rinse with cold water, or plunge into a pan of cold water. (Livers and broccoli can be cooked at the same time.) Peel and chop shallots; there should be ½ cup. Heat butter in a skillet and sauté shallots and broccoli together until shallots are translucent. Add livers and capers. While they cook, pour wine into a cup and stir in mustard. Pour over livers, and add parsley and dill. Mix well, cover the pan, and cook over low heat for 3 minutes. Serve with plain rice.

VARIATIONS: Add mushrooms, or other green vegetables. Asparagus and zucchini are good, and so are green or red peppers.

CHICKEN LIVERS PHILLIPO

TIME: 15 MINUTES
SERVINGS: 4
CALORIES: 280 PER SERVING

    1 pound fresh chicken livers
       salt
    ½ pound zucchini
    6 fresh mushrooms
    2 white onions, 1½ ounces each
    ½ pound fresh plum tomatoes, or 1 cup canned plum tomatoes
    2 tablespoons vegetable oil
    1 garlic clove, peeled
    ⅓ cup chopped fresh Italian parsley
    ¼ teaspoon Italian seasoning

Rinse livers, trim if necessary, and put in a saucepan. Cover with cold water, add a pinch of salt, and bring to a boil. Reduce heat and simmer livers for 3 minutes. Drain livers, and cut each one into 2 or 3 pieces. Wash and trim zucchini, and chop; there should be 1 cup. Wash and trim mushrooms, and chop; there should be ½ cup. Peel and chop onions. Wash fresh tomatoes, discard hard portion near stem, and chop; there should be 1 cup. If you use canned tomatoes, crush them with a wooden spoon. Heat oil in a skillet and push garlic through a press into the oil. Add zucchini, mushrooms, onions and half of the parsley, and sauté until onions are translucent and other vegetables soft. Add tomatoes and Italian seasoning and cook for a few minutes. Mash the tomatoes into the mixture. Add livers and remaining parsley and simmer for 3 minutes, or until livers are done to your taste.

QUAIL

Quails are so tiny that the usual serving per person is two. When dressed, without head, feathers and viscera, a quail weighs 4 to 4½ ounces; nearly 2 ounces of this is bones, which are not eaten. Unless you shoot your own, quails are frozen; let them defrost, still wrapped, in the refrigerator overnight. Pull off the skin or not as you prefer. Quails have very little fat, so they dry out quickly after defrosting.

QUAILS IN WHITE-WINE SAUCE

TIME: 20 MINUTES
SERVINGS: 4
CALORIES: 215 PER SERVING

2 tablespoons vegetable oil
2 garlic cloves, peeled
4 shallots, peeled
¼ cup sliced fresh mushrooms
5 tablespoons chopped fresh Italian parsley
8 quails, dressed
½ cup dry white wine
¼ teaspoon Italian seasoning
  salt and pepper

Use a pot large enough to hold all the quails. Heat the oil in the pot and push garlic through a press into the oil. Chop shallots into the pan and add mushrooms and half of the parsley. Sauté for about 2 minutes, until shallots are translucent. Add quails and brown on all sides for about 5 minutes. Add wine, Italian seasoning, and salt and pepper to taste. Cover and cook for 10 minutes. Sprinkle with remaining parsley and serve.

VARIATIONS: To thicken the sauce, mix 1 tablespoon cornstarch with 2 tablespoons cold water, and stir this slurry into the sauce after quails are transferred to a serving platter. Cook for 1 minute, stirring, and spoon over the quails.

For a more intense mushroom flavor, use about ½ ounce dried black mushrooms instead of fresh mushrooms. Soak and prepare them as described in the recipe for Mushroom Risotto (p. 94).

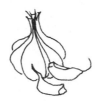

QUAILS ALLA SILVESTRO

TIME: 20 MINUTES
SERVINGS: 4
CALORIES: 225 PER SERVING

- 2 tablespoons vegetable oil
- 4 shallots, peeled
- 8 quails, dressed
- ½ pound fresh plum tomatoes
- 4 juniper berries, crushed in a mortar
- ½ cup dry red wine
- 3 tablespoons chopped fresh Italian parsley
- 1 bay leaf
   salt and pepper

Use a pot large enough to hold all the quails. Heat the oil in the pot and chop shallots into the oil. When shallots are translucent, add the quails and brown on all sides for about 5 minutes. While quails are browning, wash tomatoes and remove hard portion near stem. Chop tomatoes; there should be 1 cup. Add juniper berries and wine to quails and cook for 2 minutes. Add chopped tomatoes, parsley and bay leaf. Cover, and cook for 10 minutes. Remove bay leaf and season with salt and pepper to taste. Serve with *risotto* or polenta.

RABBIT CACCIATORA GUIDO

TIME: 25 TO 30 MINUTES
SERVINGS: 6
CALORIES: 235 PER SERVING

   2 ½ *pounds rabbit, cut into small pieces*
   1 *onion, 3 ounces*
   1 *small green pepper*
   2 *tablespoons vegetable oil*
   2 *garlic cloves, peeled*
   ½ *cup dry red wine*
   3 *tablespoons chopped fresh Italian parsley*
   ¼ *teaspoon Italian seasoning*
      salt and pepper

Rinse rabbit pieces and pat dry. (If rabbit is frozen, it should be completely defrosted before you start.) Peel and chop onion. Wash and trim green pepper, discard ribs and seeds, and chop pepper. Heat oil in a large skillet and push garlic through a press into the oil. Add chopped onion and pepper, and sauté until onion is translucent. Add rabbit pieces and sauté on all sides until browned, about 6 minutes. Add wine, parsley, Italian seasoning, and salt and pepper to taste. Cook for 10 minutes longer, until rabbit is tender.

RABBIT CACCIATORA MONICA

TIME: 25 MINUTES
SERVINGS: 6
CALORIES: 240 PER SERVING

   2 ½ *pounds rabbit, cut into small pieces*
   1 *onion, 2 ounces*
   ½ *pound fresh plum tomatoes*
   2 *ounces fresh mushrooms*
   2 *tablespoons vegetable oil*
   3 *shallots, peeled*
   ⅓ *cup chopped fresh Italian parsley*
   ¼ *teaspoon Italian seasoning*
      salt and pepper

Rinse rabbit pieces and pat dry. (If rabbit is frozen, it should be completely defrosted before you start.) Peel and chop onion. Wash tomatoes, remove hard portion near stem, and chop; there should be 1 cup. Set in a strainer to drain excess liquid. Wash and trim mushrooms, and chop; there should be ½ cup. Heat oil in a large skillet and chop shallots into the oil. Add onion and mushrooms and sauté until onion and shallots are translucent. Add rabbit pieces and sauté on all sides until browned, about 6 minutes. Add tomatoes, parsley and Italian seasoning, cover, and cook for 10 minutes, until rabbit is tender. Season the sauce with salt and pepper to taste. Serve rabbit with pasta, with the *cacciatora* sauce spooned over the pasta.

VARIATION: Use ¼ cup (about ½ ounce) dried black mushrooms instead of fresh mushrooms. Soak and prepare them as described in the recipe for Mushroom Risotto (p. 93).

RABBIT ALLA GIUSEPPE RUSSO

TIME: 35 MINUTES, EXCLUDING TIME FOR MARINATING
SERVINGS: 6
CALORIES: 215 PER SERVING

> 2½ *pounds rabbit*
> 1 *cup dry red wine*
> ¼ *cup red-wine vinegar*
> 2 *garlic cloves, peeled*
> ¼ *cup minced fresh Italian parsley*
> 3 *tablespoons minced fresh basil*
> ⅓ *teaspoon crumbled dried orégano*
> 2 *teaspoons fresh rosemary, or 1 teaspoon crushed dried rosemary*

Cut rabbit into serving pieces, rinse, and pat dry. (If rabbit is frozen, it should be completely defrosted before you start.) Arrange the pieces in a pottery or glass container that will just hold them. Pour in the wine and vinegar. Push garlic through a press into the mixture and add parsley, basil and orégano. Mix liquid and herbs and turn rabbit pieces in the marinade until all are coated. Let rabbit marinate for 30 minutes or, better, for several hours.

Transfer rabbit pieces in one layer to a shallow baking dish, and sprinkle with remaining marinade. Scatter rosemary over the top. Bake in a

preheated 350°F. oven for 30 minutes, or until done to your taste. Or broil
the rabbit about 5 inches from the source of heat. Sprinkle it with marinade
during broiling, and turn the pieces to cook twice on each side, until all test
done.

BEEF

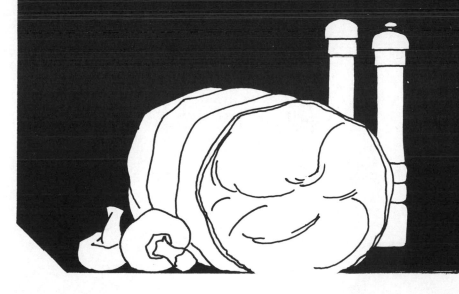

Beef plays a very small role in the Italian diet and kitchen. Cattle are hard to raise in Italy because of the lack of grazing area, and the meat is not as tasty there as in America. However, some special beef can be found around Florence and in southern Italy, and it is preferred by those who do eat beef. Nevertheless, there are in this chapter quite a few recipes for beef, because beef counts for more than 60 percent of the meat eaten in the United States. The recipes were developed from Italian classics or newly invented for low-calorie cooking. The amount of beef per serving may seem small (there are no 1-pound steaks per person to be found here), but it is adequate, and these dishes will be filling as part of a well-balanced meal with other courses.

In Italy a beefsteak is usually cut thin and often is pounded to make it even thinner. Such a thin steak is not always broiled, but is more likely to be sautéed or panfried, with wine, lemon juice and herbs. A typical recipe is Bistecca alla Fiorentina (p. 152).

Veal is naturally more popular in a country with limited grazing, and to many Italians its lighter and more delicate taste is greatly preferred to the taste of beef. In the United States in the last few years beef has been slaughtered at a younger age to save animal feeds. This younger beef is closer in texture to veal and can be cooked by the same quick methods used for veal with good results. All the recipes in the veal chapter can be adapted for young beef if beef is your preference. But we hope you will investigate the recipes for veal, which is naturally low in calories because it comes from young animals.

STEAK ALLA RITA

TIME: 10 MINUTES
SERVINGS: 4
CALORIES: 265 PER SERVING

> 1 tablespoon unsalted butter
> 4 pieces of lean beefsteak, 4 ounces each
>   salt and pepper
> 1 large lemon
> ½ cup dry white wine
> 3 tablespoons chopped fresh Italian parsley

Heat butter in a large skillet, and quickly brown the steaks on one side. Turn over, and season the browned side with salt and pepper. When underside is browned, turn again and season that side. Cut 4 thin slices from the lemon, and extract the juice from the rest. Slash steaks in the center and check for degree of pinkness you prefer. Pour the wine over steaks, reduce heat, and cook until steaks are medium-rare. At once pour lemon juice over steaks. Serve at once, with a lemon slice on each steak and parsley sprinkled over them.

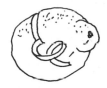

BISTECCA ALLA HENRI

TIME: 10 MINUTES
SERVINGS: 4
CALORIES: 345 PER SERVING

⅓ cup grated Parmesan cheese
6 tablespoons chopped fresh Italian parsley
   salt and pepper
4 pieces of lean beefsteak, 4 ounces each
2 tablespoons olive oil
1 garlic clove, peeled
½ cup dry red wine

Mix cheese with 3 tablespoons parsley, a pinch of salt and a little pepper, and spread on a sheet of wax paper. Press each steak into cheese mixture to coat both sides. Heat oil in a large skillet and push garlic through a press into the oil. Sauté steaks for 2 to 3 minutes per side, until lightly browned. Slash steaks in the center to check on degree of pinkness. Add wine and simmer until steaks are done to your taste. Serve with the rest of the parsley sprinkled over.

ALBERTO'S STEAK

TIME: 15 MINUTES
SERVINGS: 4
CALORIES: 335 PER SERVING

1 onion, 4 ounces
2 green peppers
2 tablespoons vegetable oil
1 garlic clove, peeled
4 pieces of lean beefsteak, 4 ounces each
½ cup dry red wine
½ teaspoon Italian seasoning
  salt and pepper
1 cup Tomato Sauce (p. 000)

Peel and chop onion. Wash peppers, remove stems, ribs and seeds, and chop peppers. Heat oil in a large skillet and push garlic through a press into the oil. Add chopped onion and peppers, and sauté until onion is translucent. Push vegetables to one side and add steaks; sauté until browned on both sides. Pour in wine, add Italian seasoning, and sprinkle steaks with salt and freshly ground pepper. Simmer for 2 minutes, then add tomato sauce and simmer until sauce is hot and steaks done to your taste.

STEAK FRANCO

TIME: 10 MINUTES
SERVINGS: 4
CALORIES: 270 PER SERVING

1 tablespoon unsalted butter
3 shallots, peeled
4 pieces of lean beefsteak, 4 ounces each
½ cup dry red wine
1 teaspoon minced fresh basil
  salt and pepper

Melt butter in a skillet and chop shallots into the pan. Sauté until shallots are translucent. Add steaks and sauté for 2 minutes on each side. Add wine and cook for 3 minutes. Add basil, and season steaks with salt and pepper. Mix sauce to distribute basil, and simmer for 1 minute. Serve with rice, with the sauce spooned over.

STEAK SALADINE

This method will result in a tender, delicious steak, even using less-expensive cuts of beef than the examples listed.

TIME: 10 MINUTES
SERVINGS: 4
CALORIES: 325 PER SERVING

      4 *pieces of beef sirloin, top round, or eye round, 4 ounces each*
      1 *tablespoon unsalted butter*
      1 *tablespoon vegetable oil*
      3 *tablespoons prepared Dijon mustard*
      ½ *cup dry red wine*
          salt and pepper
      3 *tablespoons Cognac*

Pound beef pieces flat. Heat butter and oil in a large skillet or flambé pan. Add beef and brown quickly on one side. Turn over, and spread browned sides with half of the mustard. When underside is browned, turn over again and spread second side with remaining mustard. Pour in wine and reduce heat to medium-low. Sprinkle salt and pepper over beef. Slash pieces in the center and check for degree of pinkness you prefer. Do not overcook steaks; they are best medium-rare. Heat Cognac and pour it over steaks for last minute of cooking. Ignite, and let the flame burn out naturally. Serve at once, with the sauce spooned over steaks.

Larger steaks can be prepared in the same way, but will be more caloric.

BEEFSTEAK PIAZZIOLA

TIME: 10 TO 15 MINUTES
SERVINGS: 4
CALORIES: 310 PER SERVING

    4 pieces of lean beefsteak, 4 ounces each
    ½ pound fresh plum tomatoes
    1 white onion, 1 ½ ounces
    2 tablespoons olive oil
    2 garlic cloves, peeled
    ¼ cup tomato paste
    ¼ cup chopped fresh Italian parsley
    ¼ teaspoon crumbled dried orégano
       salt and pepper

Pound steaks flat. Wash tomatoes, remove hard portion near stem, and chop; there should be 1 cup. Peel and chop onion. Heat oil in a large skillet and push garlic through a press into the oil. Add onion and sauté until translucent. Add steaks and sauté for 2 minutes. Turn steaks over. Add tomatoes, tomato paste, herbs, and salt and pepper to taste. Cook for 5 minutes. Slash steaks across center to check on degree of pinkness. Serve as soon as steaks are done to your taste.

BISTECCA ALLA FIORENTINA

TIME: 10 MINUTES
SERVINGS: 4
CALORIES: 325 PER SERVING

    4 slices of beef filet (tournedos), 4 ounces each
    3 tablespoons red Chianti wine
    2 tablespoons olive oil
    2 garlic cloves, peeled
       pinch of dried rosemary
       salt and pepper
    1 lemon, cut into very thin slices

Pound the steaks to flatten them like veal scallops. Use a shallow bowl large enough to hold the steaks, and mix in it the wine and oil. Push garlic through a press into the mixture, and add the rosemary. Mix well, then place steaks in the mixture and keep turning them until they are well coated. Steaks can be grilled or broiled, or panfried. If you grill or broil them, cook over brisk heat for 2 or 3 minutes on a side and keep basting with the marinade throughout. To panfry, place steaks and marinade in a very hot skillet and cook for 3 or 4 minutes on a side. Turn steaks twice and spoon marinade over each time. Sprinkle with salt and pepper to taste. Serve topped with lemon slices.

VARIATION: This can be made with *filets mignons* also, but as a *filet mignon* weighs twice as much as a *tournedos,* the calories are nearly doubled.

BEEF BRACIOLE

TIME: 15 MINUTES
SERVINGS: 6
CALORIES: 300 PER SERVING

> 6 thin slices of lean beef (round), about 4 ounces each
> 3 tablespoons olive oil
> 3 garlic cloves, peeled
> 3 shallots, peeled
> ⅓ cup chopped fresh Italian parsley
>   salt and pepper
> ½ cup dry red wine
>   chopped parsley for garnish

Flatten the beef slices with the flat side of a cleaver if you wish. Heat the oil in a large skillet and push the garlic through a press into the oil. Chop shallots into the oil, and sauté for a few minutes. Scoop out garlic and shallots and transfer to a small bowl; leave the oil in the pan. Add the parsley to the bowl, and mix. Sprinkle the beef slices with salt and pepper and divide the parsley mixture among the steaks, placing the filling in the center. Fold each steak over the filling, first one end, then the other, or roll up the steaks over the filling. Fasten each one with a wooden pick or stainless-steel skewer. Place rolls in the skillet and sauté for 5 minutes, turning to brown on all sides. Add the wine and cook until beef is tender and wine reduced by half, to a few teaspoons for each roll. Sprinkle with more parsley and serve.

BEEF SLICES ENRICO

TIME: 8 TO 10 MINUTES
SERVINGS: 6
CALORIES: 280 PER SERVING

2 *tablespoons vegetable oil*
2 *garlic cloves, peeled and crushed*
6 *thin slices of lean beef (filet or round), about 4 ounces each*
½ *cup dry red wine*
¼ *cup chopped fresh Italian parsley*
   juice of ½ lemon
   salt and freshly ground black pepper

Pour oil into a large skillet and add garlic. At once add the beef slices and sauté for a few minutes on each side. Add wine and parsley and cook for a few minutes longer. Sprinkle with lemon juice and salt and pepper to taste, and serve at once.

STEAK CRUDA

For this recipe use only very fresh beef, and grind or chop it only just before mixing and serving.

TIME: 10 MINUTES
SERVINGS: 12 AS MAIN DISH; 20 TO 24 AS FIRST COURSE
CALORIES: 245 PER MAIN-COURSE SERVING; 125 PER FIRST-COURSE
          SERVING

3 *pounds beef round*
¼ *cup dry red wine*
3 *tablespoons prepared Dijon mustard*
2 *teaspoons Worcestershire sauce*
1 *Bermuda or Spanish slicing onion, 8 ounces*
2 *anchovy fillets, drained*
2 *eggs*
3 *tablespoons capers*
   salt and pepper

Grind beef just before mixing or, better, knife-chop it to very fine bits, using a chef's knife and a sturdy chopping block. Turn into a large bowl, add wine, mustard and Worcestershire, and mix with forks until well blended. Peel and mince onion, and mince or mash anchovies. Break raw eggs into the meat, and add onion, anchovies and capers. Again mix until everything is well distributed. Add salt and freshly ground pepper, or let each person season his own portion. Serve in a bowl, or in a mound on a platter, or on individual plates. Good for a main dish for luncheon, and especially good for a first course. Steak Cruda can be served at stand-up parties if it is spread on whole-wheat or rye crackers or on vegetable dippers.

BEEF BURGERS ITALIA

TIME: 10 TO 12 MINUTES
SERVINGS: 8
CALORIES: 230 PER BURGER

2 *pounds lean beef (chuck, top sirloin, hanging tenderloin)*
¼ *cup dry red wine*
3 *tablespoons prepared Dijon mustard*
1 *large garlic clove, peeled*
1 *onion, 2 ounces*
3 *tablespoons chopped fresh Italian parsley*
  salt and pepper
2 *tablespoons vegetable oil*

Grind or chop beef just before you use it. Turn into a large bowl and pour in wine. Add mustard and push garlic through a press into the mixture. Peel and mince onion and add with the parsley. Mix with hands or wooden paddles. Add salt and pepper to taste—not too much of either. Heat oil in a large skillet. Shape the mixture into 8 patties, and sauté them over brisk heat, browning them on both sides, until done to your taste.

VARIATIONS: Add shredded cheese, chopped olives, green peppers or pimientos, or mashed anchovies.

CHARCOAL-GRILLED OR BROILED BURGERS: The heat used in grilling and broiling is more direct and more intense than the heat of sautéing. Therefore the cut of meat is important. Use hanging tenderloin, or half top sirloin and half chuck. Round alone will be too dry.

BEEF STEW MAMMA D

TIME: 25 MINUTES
SERVINGS: 8
CALORIES: 335 PER SERVING

3 *pounds boneless beef stew meat (chuck, cross-rib, top sirloin)*
1 *onion, 5 ounces*
8 *large fresh mushrooms*
3 *tablespoons vegetable oil*
¼ *cup chopped celery*
½ *cup dry red wine*
3 *tablespoons chopped fresh Italian parsley*
2 *teaspoons crumbled dried thyme*
  salt and pepper
¼ *cup beef stock*

Cut beef into 1½-inch cubes, or smaller if you prefer. Remove any fat or connective tissue. Peel and chop onion. Wash and trim mushrooms, and chop or slice them. Heat oil in a deep skillet or heavy saucepan. Add onion, mushrooms and celery, and sauté until onion is translucent. Add beef cubes and sauté them over medium to high heat, stirring the mixture to brown cubes on all sides. Add wine, parsley and thyme, and simmer for 3 minutes. Season beef lightly with salt and pepper (the amount of salt depends partly on how salty the stock is). Pour stock over beef, cover the pan, and cook for 5 minutes longer, or until beef is done to your taste. If it is not, add a little more stock and continue to simmer. Serve with rice or potatoes.

This method works well with reasonably tender beef; if you have tougher cuts, you may need to increase stock (or substitute water) and cook for 30 minutes to 1 hour after adding stock.

BEEF LIVER

Beef liver has a more pronounced taste than calf's liver, since it comes from an older animal, but it is just as tender and needs only brief cooking. Liver is our best source of iron and an excellent source of vitamin A. Ask your butcher for liver from young beef, and have him cut it for you when you buy it. (Precut liver dries out rapidly.) Plan to cook it within a day.

Liver cooked according to these recipes is delicious; in each case another flavor accent counteracts the beefy taste. The recipes work equally well for calf's liver.

BEEF LIVER IN EGG-YOLK SAUCE

TIME: 10 MINUTES
SERVINGS: 4
CALORIES: 300 PER SERVING

   1 *pound beef liver*
   2 *tablespoons unsalted butter*
   2 *hard-cooked egg yolks*
   ½ *tablespoon prepared Dijon mustard*
   ¼ *cup dry Marsala wine*
      salt and pepper

Peel any membranes from the liver, and cut into thin strips. Melt butter in a skillet and quickly sauté liver strips on both sides. Mash egg yolks and mix with mustard and wine. Pour over the liver and cook for 5 minutes. Add salt and pepper to taste. Serve at once.

BEEF LIVER MARSALA

TIME: 15 MINUTES
SERVINGS: 4
CALORIES: 300 PER SERVING

   1 *pound beef liver*
   1 *onion, 4 ounces*
   6 *large fresh mushrooms*
   2 *tablespoons unsalted butter*
   ½ *cup dry Marsala wine*
      salt and pepper

Peel any membranes from the liver and cut into bite-size cubes. Peel and chop onion. Wash and trim mushrooms and slice or chop them. Melt butter in a skillet and sauté onion and mushrooms for 2 minutes. Add liver and stir and cook for 3 minutes. Add Marsala, season with salt and pepper to taste, and simmer for 5 minutes, until liver is done to your taste.

BEEF LIVER AND VEGETABLES

TIME: 15 MINUTES
SERVINGS: 4
CALORIES: 280 PER SERVING

> *1 pound beef liver*
> *1 onion, 2 ounces*
> *1 zucchini, 6 ounces*
> *8 ounces canned peeled plum tomatoes*
> *2 tablespoons vegetable oil*
> *½ teaspoon Italian seasoning*
>   *salt and pepper*

Peel any membranes from the liver and cut into bite-size cubes. Peel and chop onion. Wash and trim zucchini, and chop. Drain the tomatoes (use the juices for stock or soup). Heat the oil in a skillet and sauté onion and zucchini until onion is translucent. Add liver dice and sauté for 3 minutes. Dump in the tomatoes and break them up with a wooden spoon while mixing everything together. Add Italian seasoning and cook for 5 minutes, until liver is done to your taste. Season with salt and pepper.

LIVER IN SWEET-AND-SOUR SAUCE ALLA RUSSO

TIME: 15 MINUTES
SERVINGS: 4
CALORIES: 290 PER SERVING

> *1 pound beef liver*
> *10 to 12 shallots*
> *2 tablespoons vegetable oil*
> *2 garlic cloves, peeled*
> *3 tablespoons red-wine vinegar*
> *½ teaspoon sugar*
> *2 tablespoons dark raisins*
>   *salt and pepper*

Peel any membranes from the liver and cut liver into small dice. Peel and chop shallots; there should be ½ cup. Heat oil in a skillet and push garlic through a press into the oil. Add shallots and sauté until they are translucent. Add liver dice and sauté, tossing to brown all sides. Mix vinegar and sugar in a cup and stir until sugar is dissolved; this can be done over low heat if necessary to save time. Pour vinegar into the liver and cook for 6 minutes. Add raisins and cook for 2 or 3 minutes longer. Add a little salt and pepper if necessary. Serve without delay.

LAMB

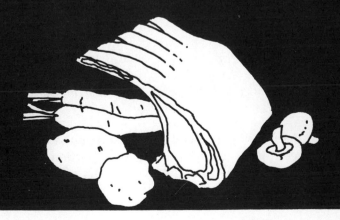

Lamb is a popular meat in Italy. It has a more distinctive taste there than in America, because of the feed, which usually includes flavorful herbs growing in the grazing areas. Young lamb is the favorite; it is tender, with little fat, and it is considered a delicacy.

In comparison to beef, lamb, being young, is not treated by the packer with any tenderizing ingredient as beef often is. Also, young lamb, which is not fatty, is much less caloric than beef. However, lamb does not have the delicate taste and texture of veal, which makes it possible to cook veal with a great variety of sauces and accompaniments.

Because of the definite flavor of lamb, there are certain herbs, spices and sauces that seem just right to enhance the taste of the meat. Rosemary and garlic are first choice. A favorite method of preparing lamb in Italy is to broil or grill it with rosemary, garlic and onions, basting with white wine, and to accompany it with potatoes. This can be done in the oven too.

Another favorite is *abbacchio,* which is a Roman dish. This is lamb roasted in the oven with vegetables and wine sauce. Skewered lamb, with vegetables also on the spit, is another favorite.

When buying lamb, look for the smallest size of whatever cut you want; it will be the youngest and the leanest.

LAMB IN OKRA-TOMATO SAUCE

TIME: 20 MINUTES
SERVINGS: 6
CALORIES: 380 PER SERVING

2   *pounds lamb cubes from shoulder or leg*
½   *pound fresh plum tomatoes*
1   *tablespoon vegetable oil*
2   *shallots, peeled*
1   *garlic clove, peeled*
2   *tablespoons Italian seasoning*
½   *pound fresh okra*
    black pepper
¼   *cup cheese (grated Parmesan, shredded mozzarella or skim-milk ricotta)*

Cut all fat off the lamb, and flatten the cubes with the flat side of a cleaver to give thin pieces. Wash tomatoes, cut out hard portion near stem, peel, and chop; there should be 1 cup. Pour the oil into a large frying pan with a cover.

Chop shallots and garlic into the pan. Add Italian seasoning and lamb pieces and sauté over brisk heat until lamb pieces are lightly browned. Add chopped tomatoes and simmer for a few minutes. Meanwhile wash okra carefully, cut off the little caps at the stem ends, and chop into ½-inch pieces. Add okra pieces to the pan with black pepper to taste, and cook for 3 minutes longer. Spoon into a 6-cup casserole dish, spoon cheese on top, and bake in a preheated 350°F. oven for 12 minutes. Or continue cooking in the frying pan; add the cheese, cover the pan, and cook for 8 minutes.

NOTE: Meat labeled "lamb stew" can come from shoulder or leg, but may also come from the neck, flank or breast. For lean pieces try to buy shoulder or leg so you can be sure to have boneless lean cubes that will cook quickly. Both portions are flavorful, but the leg will generally cost more.

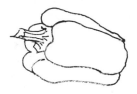

LAMB IN TOMATO SAUCE

TIME: 20 MINUTES
SERVINGS: 6
CALORIES: 400 PER SERVING

 2 *pounds lamb cubes from shoulder or leg*
 3 *tablespoons vegetable oil*
 1 *large onion, peeled and chopped*
 2 *medium-size green peppers, trimmed and chopped*
 ½ *cup dry red wine*
 1 *teaspoon Italian seasoning*
 ½ *pound fresh plum tomatoes*

Flatten the lamb cubes slightly with the flat side of a cleaver. Heat the oil in a large skillet and add chopped onion and green peppers. Sauté until onion is translucent. Add lamb cubes and sauté for 5 minutes. Add wine and Italian seasoning and cook for 2 minutes. Wash tomatoes, cut out hard portion near stem, and chop; there should be 1 cup. Drain them; the juices can be used for soups. Add chopped tomatoes, cover the skillet, and cook for 5 minutes longer, until lamb is tender and sauce well mixed.

BRAISED LAMB IN WINE

TIME: 20 MINUTES
SERVINGS: 6
CALORIES: 350 PER SERVING

2 *pounds lamb cubes from shoulder or leg*
1 *tablespoon vegetable oil*
3 *shallots, peeled*
1 *garlic clove, peeled*
3 *tablespoons minced fresh Italian parsley*
½ *cup dry red wine*
1 *tablespoon Italian seasoning*
   black pepper

Cut all fat off the lamb, and flatten the cubes with the flat side of a cleaver to give thin pieces. Pour oil into a large frying pan with a cover. Chop shallots into the pan and push garlic through a press into the pan. Add the parsley and the flattened pieces of lamb. Sauté over brisk heat until lamb pieces are lightly browned on both sides. Add the wine and Italian seasoning and bring to a boil over high heat. Reduce to barely simmering, cover, and braise for 8 to 10 minutes, until lamb is tender and done to your taste. Add more Italian seasoning if needed and black pepper to taste before serving.

BRAISED LAMB WITH GREEN BEANS

TIME: 25 MINUTES
SERVINGS: 6
CALORIES: 400 PER SERVING

2 *pounds lamb cubes from shoulder or leg*
1 *pound fresh green beans*
3 *tablespoons vegetable oil*
1 *large onion, peeled and chopped*
6 *mushrooms, sliced*
½ *cup dry white wine*
½ *teaspoon minced fresh sage*

Flatten the lamb cubes slightly with the flat side of a cleaver. Wash and trim the beans, and steam them for 8 minutes; drain and cool them. Heat the oil in a large skillet over medium heat. Add lamb pieces and sauté, tossing the pieces to brown both sides in the hot oil. Add chopped onion and sliced mushrooms. Chop steamed green beans and add to lamb. Pour in the wine and add the sage. Cover the pan and braise the lamb for 10 minutes, or until cooked to your taste.

AGNELLO IN SPIEDINI
Lamb on Skewers

TIME: 15 MINUTES
SERVINGS: 6
CALORIES: 375 PER SERVING

2 *pounds lamb shoulder*
1 *tablespoon vegetable oil*
4 *shallots, peeled*
¼ *cup tomato paste*
¼ *cup chopped fresh Italian parsley*
3 *tablespoons grated Parmesan cheese*
¼ *teaspoon ground sage*
3 *juniper berries, crushed in a mortar*
½ *cup dry red wine*

Cut lamb into pieces 1 by 1 by 2 inches; trim away all fat and any sinews. Heat oil in a skillet, and chop shallots into the oil. Add lamb pieces and brown on both sides. Drain pieces on paper towels. In a bowl mix tomato paste, parsley, cheese, sage and juniper berries to make a thick paste. Drain shallots from skillet and add to paste if you like. Thread the lamb pieces on 6 skewers and spread the paste over the pieces. Grill over a hot barbecue or broil in a preheated broiler. Baste with red wine during grilling so lamb does not dry out. Turn to cook both sides. Lamb is most flavorful when still somewhat pink in the center, but continue to cook until done to your taste.

VARIATION: If you lack grill or broiler, the coated pieces can be finished in the skillet. First pour off most of the fat in the skillet. Baste lamb with the wine and cook until tender.

LAMB CHOPS BANFI

TIME: 15 MINUTES
SERVINGS: 6
CALORIES: 210 PER SERVING

2 tablespoons vegetable oil
1 small onion, peeled and chopped
6 lamb rib chops, 5 ounces each, well trimmed
½ cup dry red wine
1 teaspoon minced fresh rosemary, or ½ teaspoon dried
½ teaspoon minced fresh sage
  salt and pepper

Heat oil in a large skillet, add onion, and sauté until onion is translucent. Add chops and sauté until lightly browned on both sides. Add wine, herbs, and salt and pepper to taste. Cover, and braise for 6 minutes.

BRAISED LAMB CHOPS WITH MIXED VEGETABLES

TIME: 25 TO 30 MINUTES
SERVINGS: 4
CALORIES: 350 PER SERVING

4 lamb shoulder chops, 7 ounces each
8 to 10 shallots
1 large green pepper
6 celery ribs with leaves
6 fresh plum tomatoes
2 tablespoons vegetable oil
2 garlic cloves, peeled
1 teaspoon minced fresh basil
¼ cup chopped fresh Italian parsley
  salt and pepper
¼ cup dry red wine

Trim chops of fat, and notch the membranes around the edges so chops will not curl up during cooking. Peel and mince shallots. Wash and trim green pepper, discard ribs and seeds, and chop pepper. Slice celery, including leaves. Wash tomatoes, remove hard portion around stem, and chop. Heat oil in a skillet large enough to hold chops in a single layer, and push garlic through a press into the oil. Sauté for 1 minute, then quickly brown chops on both sides. Transfer chops to a plate. Put shallots, green pepper and celery in the skillet and sauté until shallots are translucent. Add tomatoes, basil and parsley, and simmer for 10 minutes. Sprinkle chops with a little salt and pepper and return them to the pan. Pour wine over chops. Cover skillet and braise chops for 10 minutes, until done to your taste. Serve some of the vegetable mixture with each chop.

Braising can be done in the oven. Spoon vegetable mixture into a shallow baking pan, arrange chops on top, and cover. Bake in a preheated 350°F. oven for 15 minutes.

LAMB WITH PEPPERS

TIME: 20 MINUTES
SERVINGS: 4
CALORIES: 345 PER SERVING

> 4 green peppers
> 2 onions, 3 ounces each
> 2 tablespoons olive oil
> 2 garlic cloves, peeled
> 4 lamb steaks cut from the leg, 6 to 7 ounces each
>   salt and black pepper
> ½ teaspoon crumbled dried orégano
> ⅛ teaspoon crushed red pepper
> ½ cup white wine

Wash and trim peppers, discard ribs and seeds, and cut peppers into long strips no wider than ½ inch. Peel and chop onions. Heat oil in a skillet large enough to hold the steaks. Push garlic through a press into the oil and sauté for 1 minute. Sauté lamb steaks over brisk heat until lightly browned on both sides. Transfer to a plate and sprinkle lightly on both sides with salt and black pepper. Add onions to skillet and sauté until translucent. Add pepper strips and sauté, turning often, for about 5 minutes, until peppers are almost tender. Sprinkle in orégano and red pepper and pour in wine. Return steaks to the skillet, cover, and braise for 5 minutes, until lamb is done to your taste. Serve with rice.

VARIATIONS: Lamb steaks can be found in supermarkets; if not, your butcher can cut them for you. If you can't find them, lamb shoulder or blade chops are good prepared this way.

LAMB WITH MUSTARD AND LEMON

TIME: 15 MINUTES
SERVINGS: 4
CALORIES: 320 PER SERVING

> 2 tablespoons vegetable oil
> 4 lamb steaks cut from the leg, 6 to 7 ounces each
>   salt and black pepper
> ½ cup dry white wine
> 3 tablespoons prepared Dijon mustard
> 2 garlic cloves, peeled
> 2 tablespoons grated lemon rind
> ¼ cup chopped fresh Italian parsley

Heat oil in a skillet large enough to hold the steaks. Sauté steaks over brisk heat for 3 minutes on each side. Sprinkle them with salt and pepper when turning them. Meanwhile, pour wine into a small bowl and stir in mustard. Push garlic through a press into the wine and add lemon rind; mix well. Pour the mustard mixture over steaks, cover the skillet, and simmer for about 5 minutes longer, until steaks are done to your taste. The sauce mixture will thicken. If it becomes too thick, a little more wine can be added, or lemon juice. Spoon pan sauce over steaks, and sprinkle with parsley.

LAMB WITH FENNEL SAUCE

TIME: 25 TO 30 MINUTES
SERVINGS: 8
CALORIES: 410 PER SERVING

> 6 pounds leg of lamb
> 2 pounds fresh fennel
>   salt
> 2 onions, 3 ounces each
> 2 tablespoons olive oil
> 1 garlic clove, peeled
> ¼ cup tomato paste
> ⅓ teaspoon Italian seasoning
>   pepper

Cut lamb from the bones, remove all fat and skin, and cut meat into small cubes or rectangles, no thicker than 1 inch. Pull off tough outer ribs of fennel, cut off the top portions of inner ribs, and dice the hearts. Drop fennel into a pot of cold water, add a pinch of salt for each cup of the water, and bring to a boil. Reduce to a simmer and cook for a few minutes, until fennel is soft but not mushy. Drain fennel. Peel and chop onions. Heat oil in a large skillet and push garlic through a press into the oil. Add onions and sauté until onions are translucent. Add the lamb pieces and continue to sauté, turning the pieces to brown on all sides. Add tomato paste, Italian seasoning and a few tablespoons of water; the amount of water depends on the moistness of all the other ingredients. Add drained fennel and cook for 8 minutes. If mixture seems too dry, add a little more water, 1 tablespoon at a time. Stir during cooking to mix everything together. Season with salt and pepper to taste if needed.

LAMB AND VEGETABLE MISTO

TIME: 20 MINUTES
SERVINGS: 6
CALORIES: 325 PER SERVING

> 2 *pounds lamb stew meat, without fat*
> 1 *pound fresh plum tomatoes*
> 2 *tablespoons vegetable oil*
> 2 *white potatoes, 4 ounces each, peeled and diced*
> 2 *carrots, scraped and sliced thin*
> 2 *celery ribs, chopped*
> 1 *unpeeled zucchini, 10 ounces, chopped*
> 1 *white onion, 3 ounces, peeled and minced*
> 5 *shallots, peeled and minced*
> 2 *garlic cloves, peeled*
> ½ *cup dry red wine*
> ¼ *cup chopped fresh Italian parsley*
> ½ *teaspoon Italian seasoning*
>   *freshly ground black pepper*

Dice lamb stew meat, and prepare all the vegetables. Wash tomatoes, remove hard portion near stem, and chop; there should be 2 cups. Set in a strainer to drain excess liquid. Heat the oil in a large pot and add potatoes, carrots, celery, zucchini, onion and shallots. Push garlic through a press into the mixture. Mix with a wooden spoon, then sauté for 5 minutes, stirring occasionally. Add the lamb bits and brown them for a few minutes. Add red wine, stir, and cook for 1 minute. Add tomatoes, parsley, Italian seasoning, and black pepper to taste. Cover and cook for 5 minutes.

VARIATIONS: Omit potatoes, and serve the stew over brown rice.

Add mushrooms, green peppers, okra, eggplant or broccoli for quite a different taste and texture.

VEAL

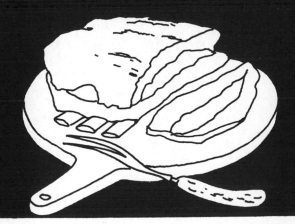

Veal is Italy's first meat. Italians prefer the taste to that of beef, and also value the fact that veal is lighter and less caloric. (Also, as we have already noted, there is relatively little beef in Italy.) Americans are beginning to select veal more and more because it is lean and naturally tender.

The texture and taste of veal is deliciously accompanied with light white-wine sauces, sweeter Marsala sauces, red-wine or tomato sauces. Many herbs and vegetables can be used. There are probably a hundred or more ways to cook *scaloppine,* the thin slices cut from the leg. Since these slices are so thin, they cook in minutes, and the amount of oil needed in the pan can be measured in teaspoons. Less than a teaspoon is needed for a single *scaloppina.*

You may find so-called *scaloppine* from various parts of the leg, even cut from the shoulder, in supermarkets, but to be just right, these should be slices cut across the round of the leg, after all membranes and veins have been removed. They are cut very thin, and usually pounded thinner. Your butcher can do this for you, or you can do it at home. Place the scallop between two sheets of wax paper and pound with the flat side of a cleaver. The wax paper keeps the surface smooth and prevents tearing of the meat. A slice about 2 by 4 inches, before pounding, will weigh about 2 ounces, which may surprise you, but remember all we've said about veal being light; it really is.

Cook these little slices over low to medium heat for 2 to 3 minutes on each side. Never overcook, and as soon as they are done remove them from heat or you will lose the light delicate texture.

If you have thicker pieces, slash the veal lengthwise after the first minutes of cooking to check the color. The minute the color goes past the pink stage to white, the veal is ready to serve. Don't cook it even a minute past that point!

Keep in mind that many sauces for fish and chicken can be used for veal, and the reverse is true also, except that Marsala is more appropriate for veal than for chicken or fish.

Be selective in buying veal. It is expensive in America, unfortunately, but it is not an economy to buy less than the best veal. If you are a novice, consult your butcher. You will find one hidden away even in supermarkets. The recipe you use can be chosen for the occasion, for your mood, or according to what's in your cupboard, because veal is the most adaptable meat you can buy.

VEAL LIMONE

TIME: 10 MINUTES
SERVINGS: 4
CALORIES: 325 PER SERVING

8 veal scallops, about 2 ounces each
2 tablespoons vegetable oil
2 shallots, peeled
½ cup dry white wine
   pinch of black pepper
3 lemons
2 teaspoons chopped fresh Italian parsley

Flatten veal scallops with the flat side of a cleaver to make a thin layer of meat. Heat the oil in a large frying pan. Chop the shallots into the pan and add the veal slices; sauté veal for 2 minutes on each side. Pour wine over the veal, and sprinkle in the pepper; cook for 2 minutes. Meanwhile extract juice from 2 lemons and cut the third into very thin slices. Remove any seeds from the slices. Add juice and slices to the veal. Stir well and cook for a few minutes longer, until everything is hot. Sprinkle with parsley. Serve hot without delay, or let the dish cool and serve cold later.

VEAL PICCATA ALLA ENRICO

TIME: 10 MINUTES
SERVINGS: 4
CALORIES: 300 PER SERVING

2 tablespoons vegetable oil
1 garlic clove, peeled
8 veal scallops, 2 ounces each
   salt and pepper
   juice of 2 lemons
3 tablespoons chopped fresh Italian parsley

Heat oil in a large skillet. Push garlic through a press into the oil and sauté for 2 minutes. Add the veal scallops and sauté for 2 minutes on each side. Add salt and pepper to taste, the lemon juice and parsley, and cook for 3 minutes longer, turning the scallops in the sauce to coat well.

VITELLO CON MOZZARELLA

TIME: 15 MINUTES
SERVINGS: 4
CALORIES: 380 PER SERVING

1 *large onion, 3 ounces*
2 *tablespoons vegetable oil*
4 *veal scallops, 4 ounces each*
½ *cup dry red wine*
1 *teaspoon Italian seasoning*
   salt and pepper
4 *slices of skim-milk mozzarella cheese, about 1 ounce each*
2 *tablespoons chopped fresh Italian parsley*

Peel and chop onion. Heat oil in a large skillet and sauté onion for 2 minutes. Add veal scallops and sauté for 3 minutes on each side. Add wine, Italian seasoning, and salt and pepper to taste. Mix well, and cook for 2 minutes. Place 1 cheese slice on each scallop, remove the pan from the heat, and cover the pan for 2 minutes. Sprinkle each scallop with parsley when serving.

VITELLO TONNATO

TIME: 15 MINUTES, EXCLUDING TIME FOR CHILLING
SERVINGS: 4
CALORIES: 350 PER SERVING

4 *ounces canned water-packed tuna*
1 *onion, 2 ounces*
2 *tablespoons vegetable oil*
8 *veal scallops, 2 ounces each*
¼ *cup dry white wine*
¼ *cup skim-milk ricotta cheese*
2 *tablespoons prepared Dijon mustard*
2 *lemons*
3 *tablespoons capers*
   salt and pepper
¼ *cup chopped fresh Italian parsley*

Drain the tuna well, then mash; set aside. Peel and chop the onion. Heat the oil in a large skillet and sauté onion for 2 minutes. Add veal scallops and sauté for 2 minutes on each side. Add wine and cook for 2 minutes. Mix together the ricotta, mustard, mashed tuna, juice of 1 lemon, capers, and salt and pepper to taste. Pour over the veal and mix well. Cook for 3 or 4 minutes. Cool, then chill. Slice remaining lemon into delicate thin slices. Serve the veal with lemon slices and chopped parsley on top.

VEAL MARSALA WITH GRAPES

TIME: 10 MINUTES
SERVINGS: 4
CALORIES: 295 PER SERVING

> 8 *veal scallops, about 2 ounces each*
> 1 *cup white grapes*
> 2 *shallots*
> ½ *teaspoon minced fresh tarragon*
> 2 *sprigs of Italian parsley*
> ½ *cup dry Marsala wine*

Flatten the veal scallops with the flat side of a cleaver to make a very thin layer of meat. Wash grapes and roll in a towel to dry completely. With a sharp knife split each grape lengthwise into halves. If there are any seeds, remove them. Place scallops in a large skillet. Peel shallots and cut into the pan. Add herbs and wine. Bring the wine to a boil, reduce to a simmer, and cook for 3 minutes on each side. Add grapes and simmer for a few minutes longer, just until fruit is heated. Discard parsley sprigs. Serve hot or cold.

This is good for simple and plain occasions, but it is also great for festive buffets.

VEAL JOSEPHIE
Veal with Lemon and Chives

TIME: 12 MINUTES
SERVINGS: 4
CALORIES: 325 PER SERVING

1 *large onion, 3 ounces*
2 *tablespoons vegetable oil*
8 *veal scallops, 2 ounces each*
   juice of 2 lemons
¼ *cup dry vermouth*
   salt and pepper
3 *tablespoons snipped fresh chives*

Peel and mince the onion. Heat oil in a large skillet, and add onion. Sauté for 2 minutes. Add veal scallops and sauté for 2 minutes on each side. Add lemon juice, vermouth, and salt and pepper to taste. Cook for 4 minutes. Sprinkle with chives and serve hot or cold.

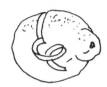

VITELLO PIETRO
Veal with Cheese and Asparagus

TIME: 15 MINUTES
SERVINGS: 4
CALORIES: 380 PER SERVING

6 *fresh asparagus*
2 *tablespoons vegetable oil*
4 *veal scallops, 4 ounces each*
½ *cup dry white wine*
1 *teaspoon Italian seasoning*
3 *tablespoons chopped fresh Italian parsley*
   salt and pepper
4 *slices of skim-milk mozzarella cheese, about 1 ounce each*

Cut off tough portion of asparagus, wash, and cut stalks into ½-inch pieces. Blanch or steam for 2 or 3 minutes, until just tender and still green. Heat oil in a large skillet and sauté veal scallops for 2 minutes on each side. Add wine, Italian seasoning, parsley, and salt and pepper to taste, and cook for a few minutes. Arrange asparagus pieces over the scallops and top each one with a slice of cheese. Cover the skillet and leave over low heat for a minute or two, until the cheese melts. Serve at once.

VEAL FLAMBÉ ENNIO
Veal in Cognac Sauce

TIME: 10 TO 12 MINUTES
SERVINGS: 4
CALORIES: 305 PER SERVING

6 fresh mushrooms
1 tablespoon unsalted butter
8 veal scallops, 2 ounces each
½ cup dry white wine
1 teaspoon crumbled dried thyme
salt and pepper
2 to 3 tablespoons Cognac

Wash and trim mushrooms and cut into thin slices. Melt the butter in a large skillet and sauté the mushrooms for 1 minute. Add the veal scallops and sauté for 2 minutes on each side. Add wine, thyme, and a tiny pinch of salt and pepper. Cook for 2 minutes. Warm the Cognac, pour it over the veal, and ignite. Let the flame burn out naturally, and serve at once.

VEAL GIORGIO
Veal with Shrimps and Asparagus

TIME: 20 MINUTES
SERVINGS: 4
CALORIES: 350 PER SERVING

8 fresh asparagus
12 small shrimps
2 tablespoons vegetable oil
1 garlic clove, peeled
3 shallots, peeled
¼ cup chopped fresh Italian parsley
8 veal scallops, about 2 ounces each
½ cup dry white wine
3 tablespoons lemon juice
salt and pepper
lemon slices or wedges

Wash and trim asparagus; discard all tough portions. Shell and devein the shrimps. Steam or blanch the asparagus for 5 minutes; it should still be green; drain. At the same time poach the shrimps for 5 minutes; drain. Heat the oil in a large skillet. Push the garlic through a press into the oil. Chop shallots into the oil and add the parsley. Sauté until shallots are translucent, then add the veal scallops and sauté for 2 minutes on each side. Remove veal to a serving platter or individual plates, and keep warm. Put drained asparagus and shrimps in the skillet, and add wine, lemon juice, and salt and pepper to taste. Cook for a few minutes, then arrange 2 asparagus stalks and 3 shrimps on each veal scallop and spoon the sauce over all. Garnish with more lemon—slices or wedges.

VEAL SCALOPPINE ALLA PALMA

TIME: 15 MINUTES
SERVINGS: 4
CALORIES: 375 PER SERVING

8 *veal scallops, about 2 ounces each*
½ *cup grated Parmesan cheese*
½ *cup minced fresh Italian parsley*
1 *tablespoon unsalted butter*
1 *tablespoon olive oil*
½ *cup dry white wine*

Pound veal scallops with the flat side of a cleaver to make thin layers of meat. Mix cheese and parsley on a board or sheet of wax paper. Press each scallop into the mixture on both sides and press firmly to coat well. Let the scallops rest on another sheet of wax paper until ready to cook. Melt butter with oil in a large skillet. Sauté veal slices in a single layer for about 3 minutes a side; do them in several batches if necessary rather than crowding them. Return all scallops to the pan and add the wine. Simmer for a few minutes, then serve at once.

VEAL ROLLS

TIME: 20 MINUTES
SERVINGS: 4
CALORIES: 380 PER SERVING

     8 *veal scallops, about 2 ounces each*
     2 *tablespoons vegetable oil*
     ½ *cup shredded skim-milk mozzarella cheese*
     ¼ *cup chopped fresh mushrooms*
     ¼ *cup chopped fresh Italian parsley*
     ½ *cup dry white wine*
     1 *tablespoon prepared Dijon mustard*
        dash of black pepper
     1 *teaspoon Italian seasoning*
        salt

Flatten veal scallops with the flat side of a cleaver to make a very thin layer of meat. Heat the oil in a large frying pan and sauté the veal slices, a few at a time, for 2 minutes on each side. Remove slices from oil and drain; pat dry and arrange in a row on your work surface. Use the oil left in the pan to oil a baking dish large enough to hold the rolls in a single layer; a shallow oval baker about 8 by 6 inches is a good size. Mix cheese, mushrooms and parsley, and divide the mixture among the veal slices, placing it in the middle of each scallop. Roll up the slices and press tightly to seal, or fasten with a tiny stainless-steel skewer. Place the rolls in the baking dish.

    Pour the wine into a small saucepan. Add mustard, pepper, Italian seasoning, and salt to taste. Bring to a boil over low heat, and stir to mix well. Pour the sauce over the veal rolls, and bake in a preheated 400°F. oven for 10 minutes.

VARIATIONS: A change in the filling will make the dish very different. Instead of mushrooms, try chopped shrimps, or onions, or zucchini, or Italian peppers. Instead of mozzarella, use skim-milk ricotta.

VEAL AND PEPPERS LUIGI

TIME: 20 MINUTES
SERVINGS: 4
CALORIES: 400 PER SERVING

    4 veal loin chops, 6 ounces each
    1 large onion, 3 ounces
    3 green peppers
    1 pound fresh plum tomatoes, or canned whole plum tomatoes
    3 tablespoons vegetable oil
    ½ cup dry red wine
    2 teaspoons crushed dried orégano
    ½ teaspoon crushed red pepper
    salt and pepper

Have the chops pounded flat. They can be boned or not as you prefer. Peel onion and slice into thin shreds. Wash peppers, remove ribs and all seeds, and cut peppers into slivers. Wash tomatoes, chop, and drain; or drain the canned tomatoes. Heat the oil in a large skillet and sauté onion and peppers for about 3 minutes. Add veal chops and brown on both sides. Add wine, orégano, red pepper, and salt and pepper to taste. Cook for 2 minutes. Add the chopped fresh tomatoes or the canned tomatoes. Break up the canned tomatoes with a spoon as they cook. Simmer, stirring often, for 5 minutes. Serve hot.

VARIATIONS: Bone the chops and cut the meat into bite-size pieces.

    Add mushrooms, chopped or sliced, when sautéing the onions and peppers.

    For a spicier taste, add more red pepper.

VEAL CHOPS WITH ROSEMARY

      TIME: 12 TO 15 MINUTES
SERVINGS: 4
CALORIES: 325 PER SERVING

    2 tablespoons olive oil
    1 garlic clove, peeled
    4 veal loin chops, 6 ounces each
    ½ cup dry red wine
    2 teaspoons crumbled dried rosemary
    salt and pepper

Heat the oil in a large skillet. Push the garlic through a press into the oil and cook for 2 minutes. Add chops and sauté until lightly browned on both sides. Add wine, rosemary, and a pinch of salt and pepper. Turn the chops in the herbed wine and cook for 2 minutes.

VEAL CHOPS SASSI
Veal Chops with Artichokes

TIME: 20 MINUTES, EXCLUDING TIME TO COOK AND COOL
ARTICHOKES
SERVINGS: 6
CALORIES: 275 PER SERVING

4 *large artichoke bottoms, cooked (p. 195) and cooled*
3 *tablespoons olive oil*
4 *shallots, peeled*
2 *garlic cloves, peeled*
¼ *cup chopped fresh Italian parsley*
6 *veal loin chops, 6 ounces each*
  salt and pepper
½ *cup dry red wine*
¼ *cup brandy*

Remove any leaves and the chokes from artichokes, and cut the bottoms into large dice. Heat the oil in a large skillet. Chop shallots into the oil and push the garlic through a press into the pan. Add half of the parsley and sauté until shallots are translucent. Add the chops and sauté them in the oil for 2 minutes on each side. Sprinkle chops lightly with salt and pepper. Add wine and diced artichoke, cover, and cook for 5 minutes, or until chops are cooked to your taste. Transfer chops to a serving platter and sprinkle them with the rest of the parsley. With a slotted spoon lift out the artichoke dice and arrange them around the chops. Warm the brandy in a small saucepan, then ignite it and pour it flaming into the skillet. When flames die out naturally, pour the sauce over the chops. Serve at once, with braised small potatoes.

VEAL GENOVESE ADELAIDE
Veal with Shallots and White Wine

TIME: 40 MINUTES
SERVINGS: 8 (2 SLICES EACH)
CALORIES: 215 PER SERVING

2 pounds boneless veal shoulder
2 white onions, 1 ½ ounces each
8 to 10 shallots
¼ cup chopped fresh Italian parsley
½ cup veal stock
½ cup dry white wine

Tie the veal in a narrow compact roll, with pieces of white string about 1 inch apart crosswise and a single string lengthwise. Peel onions and cut into strips from top to bottom. Peel and mince shallots; there should be ⅓ cup. Place onions, shallots and parsley in a heavy pot with a cover just large enough to hold the meat. (If pot is too large the meat will steam instead of braising.) Arrange the veal on the vegetable bed and pour in stock and wine. Bring to a boil, then reduce to a simmer, cover, and simmer for 30 minutes, or until veal is nearly done to your taste. Lift the meat from the pan and cut and remove the strings. Return to the pan and simmer for a few minutes longer. Remove veal to a platter or carving board and cut into very thin slices. Serve the cooking liquids as a sauce; to make a smooth sauce, purée the whole mixture in an electric blender.

FEGATO ALLA CORRINE
Calf's Liver with Marsala

TIME: 10 MINUTES
SERVINGS: 4
CALORIES: 180 PER SERVING

1 pound calf's liver
¼ pound white onions
2 tablespoons unsalted butter
½ cup sweet Marsala wine
salt and pepper
¼ cup chopped fresh Italian parsley

Remove all membranes from liver and cut into very thin slices. Peel and chop white onions; there should be ½ cup. Melt butter in a skillet and sauté onions until translucent. Add liver slices and sauté for 1 minute on each side. Add wine and cook for 4 minutes. Season to taste, add parsley, and serve without delay.

FEGATO ALLA VENEZIANA

TIME: 10 MINUTES
SERVINGS: 4
CALORIES: 145 PER SERVING

> 1 *pound calf's liver*
> 1 *onion, 4 ounces*
> 1 *tablespoon unsalted butter*
> 1 *tablespoon olive oil*
> 3 *tablespoons chopped fresh Italian parsley*
> *salt and pepper*

Remove all membranes from liver and cut into very thin slices. Peel and slice the onion. Melt butter with oil in a skillet and sauté onion slices for 2 minutes. Add liver slices and sauté for 5 minutes, browning slices on both sides. Sprinkle with parsley, season to taste, and serve without delay.

EGG DISHES

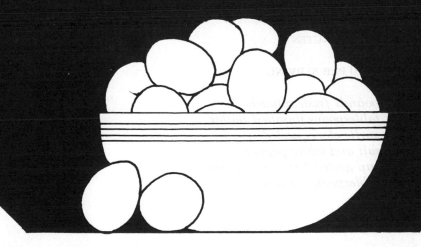

In Italy eggs are not served for breakfast; rather they are served for lunch or dinner with a variety of fillings, mainly as a first course or as a light main course.

While all traditional methods of cooking eggs are used—poached *(affogate)*, scrambled *(strapazzate)*, fried *(fritte)*, baked *(al forno)*, boiled *(bollite)*, and shirred *(cocotte)*—the most popular egg preparation is the *frittata*, a flattened omelet.

A *frittata* consists of beaten eggs combined with diced cooked vegetables, cheese, herbs, sometimes ham or seafood; but vegetables and cheese are the most popular. A *frittata* is cooked on both sides like a pancake, and is cut into wedges like a pie. A variety of sauces can be served with this flattened omelet. A quick meal can be based on a *frittata.* Serve a vegetable or seafood *frittata* with a mixed salad, cheese and fruit, with a bottle of Italian wine to accompany and complement everything.

Another great favorite made with eggs is the Italian egg pie, the *tortina*. A *tortina* is made of cooked vegetables, often combined with cheese, ham or seafood, added to beaten eggs; the mixture is poured into a pie pan, which can be lined with pastry or not, or it can be poured over bread slices; it is then baked in the oven. A *tortina* can be served hot or cold, with sauces, or just sprinkled with Parmesan cheese.

The *frittata* and *tortina* can be made with an enormous variety of fillings. The finished preparation can be decorated with a sauce, or the top can be arranged with sliced olives, slivered peppers or other vegetables diced—almost like decorating a pizza—to make a beautiful presentation. All egg dishes are quick and give you an opportunity for creative cookery.

EGGS FLORENTINE CARLO

TIME: 20 MINUTES
SERVINGS: 4
CALORIES: 210 PER SERVING

> 2 *pounds fresh spinach*
> 2 *tablespoons unsalted butter*
> 1 *garlic clove, peeled*
>   *salt and white pepper*
> ¼ *cup grated Parmesan cheese*
> 1 *tablespoon vegetable oil*
> 4 *eggs*

Wash spinach thoroughly, then cook in just the water clinging to the leaves for 4 minutes. Lift from the saucepan to a colander and chop; there should be about 2 cups. Melt butter over low heat and push garlic through a press into butter. Sauté for 1 minute, then add chopped spinach and sauté and turn until spinach is well buttered. Season with salt and white pepper to taste. Off the heat stir in half of the cheese. Use the oil to coat 4 shallow baking dishes that hold about 1 cup each. Divide spinach among the dishes, and make a depression in the center of each one. Break an egg into each depression and sprinkle ½ tablespoon cheese over each egg. Set the dishes in cake tins or other larger pans containing ½ inch of hot water. Bake in a preheated 350°F. oven for 12 minutes, or until the eggs are done to your taste. Yolks should still be liquid, the cheese golden.

FRITTATA

Ah, the joys of this Italian "pancake"—from cocktail food or first course to a glorious sweet dessert! It can make an entire meal, with a salad and some fruit. A *frittata* is fast, easy, light and very healthful.

It is usual to say that a *frittata* is to the Italians like an *omelette* to the French, but actually a *frittata* is more flexible. This versatile dish can be used for nearly every course. It can be used for cocktail food; cut the *frittata* into small squares and dip them into tomato, cheese or vegetable sauce. It makes an excellent first course; serve a large pie-shaped piece, just as if serving a quiche. For a first-course *frittata* mix the eggs with vegetables, seafood, chicken, meat or cheese, or prepare it just plain. Serve a *frittata* as a main course, with all the fillings mentioned for a first course, and many varieties of sauces and toppings—cheese, tomato, vegetable purées, or chopped olives, almonds or herbs. Also, prepare a *frittata* like a pizza, with the sauce and filling on top, and sprinkle with Parmesan cheese; be sure to brown both sides slightly for this style. Finally, a sweet *frittata* makes a perfect ending to a meal (see Desserts for sweet *fritatta*). A combination of fruit and cheese, all in one, is another possible recipe.

The fillings for *frittata* can be vegetables, chicken, meat, fish or cheese, one ingredient or a mixture, in any combination that suits your purpose. All ingredients should be cut into fine slices or chopped or minced. They can be used raw if the time for cooking the *frittata* is enough time to cook the filling. If the ingredients should be cooked, oil-steam them (see Broccoli all'Olio, p. 199), or blanch them in salted water, or steam them, but for a short time only;

the vegetables should be tender but crisp. Fish, chicken or meat should be tender and still moist, not dried out or overdone; they can be sautéed or poached. The possible combinations for filling are so many that you could invent a different *frittata* every week.

EGGS MIXED WITH FILLING, COOKED IN A SKILLET: Mix filling with eggs. Heat 2 tablespoons olive or vegetable oil in a heavy skillet or omelet pan. Pour in the egg mixture, making a layer about ½ inch thick. Cook on one side until set, then slide off onto an oiled pan and flip over to cook the underside. Or, when one side is set, slide the skillet under the broiler for a minute or two to finish cooking the upper side. Or, when one side is set, cover the skillet and continue to cook until the top is set.

FILLING BAKED IN THE OVEN WITH EGGS ADDED ON TOP: Arrange the filling in a baking dish and cook it in the oven for a few minutes. Beat the eggs lightly, pour them over the filling, and continue to bake until the top is set. Serve the *frittata* in the baking dish and cut it like a pie.

FRITTATA WITH SAUCE ON TOP: Sauce can be added to the *frittata* that is baked in the oven or finished in the broiler during the last few minutes of setting. Tomato or cheese sauce or a vegetable purée can be used. Other possibilities are mushrooms, sliced or chopped; chopped pitted olives; red pimientos, cut into thin strips; almonds, slivered or diced; raisins; mozzarella or Swiss cheese, cut into thin slices; or grated Parmesan cheese.

If you plan to finish cooking a *frittata* in oven or broiler, be sure to use a sturdy skillet with a heatproof handle. The classic French omelet pan is all metal, but the angle of the handle makes it awkward to use in many home broilers. It is possible to cook a *frittata* in a square or rectangular pan, and this is a good choice if you plan to use it for apéritif food—it will be easier to cut into squares.

FRITTATA

TIME: 15 MINUTES
SERVINGS: 6 FOR FIRST COURSE; 4 FOR MAIN COURSE
CALORIES: 90 PER FIRST-COURSE SERVING; 135 PER MAIN-COURSE
SERVING

1 to 2 tablespoons vegetable or olive oil
6 eggs
3 tablespoons water
5 tablespoons chopped fresh Italian parsley
¼ teaspoon Italian seasoning
½ cup filling
salt and pepper

FILLING: Anything you like; good vegetables are mushrooms, onions, green or red peppers, zucchini or other tender squashes. Cheese, alone or mixed with vegetables, is also good.

Pour enough of the oil into a large skillet to cover the bottom. Beat eggs lightly with the water, parsley and Italian seasoning. Add the filling, season with salt and pepper to taste, and blend thoroughly. Heat the pan over low to medium heat, and pour in the egg mixture, making a layer about ½ inch thick. Cook for 3 or 4 minutes, until the bottom is brown and firm. Shake the pan gently to prevent sticking. Oil a plate slightly larger than the pan. Place it upside down on the pan and, holding pan and plate firmly together, turn them over. Slide the *frittata* back into the pan with the uncooked side down. Continue to cook for a few minutes, until the underside is cooked to your taste. Turn out and serve.

Or try either of the other methods—cover the skillet and continue cooking for a few minutes to set the top; or slide the pan under the broiler and cook for a few minutes until the top is finished to your taste.

VARIATIONS: Serve with a topping of tomato sauce or cheese sauce. Serve with a vegetable mixture or purée spooned on top like *egg foo yung*.

Sprinkle with grated Parmesan cheese, or other cheese topping.

FRITTATA WITH PASTA

TIME: 10 MINUTES
SERVINGS: 6
CALORIES: 200 PER SERVING

> 6 *eggs*
> ⅓ *cup grated Parmesan cheese*
> ¼ *cup chopped fresh Italian parsley*
> ⅓ *teaspoon Italian seasoning*
> 2 *cups cooked pasta, cooked just* al dente
> 1 *tablespoon plus 1 teaspoon vegetable oil*
> ½ *cup Tomato Sauce (p. 245) or Ricotta Sauce (p. 236)*
>   *grated cheese and parsley sprigs for garnish*

Beat the eggs in a large bowl and stir in cheese, parsley, Italian seasoning and pasta; mix well. Heat 1 tablespoon oil in a skillet and pour in the *frittata* mixture. Cook for 2 or 3 minutes, until browned on the bottom. Use rest of the oil to coat a plate slightly larger than the skillet. Place it upside down on the pan and, holding pan and plate firmly together, turn them over. Slide the *frittata* back into the pan with the uncooked side down. Cook for 2 or 3 minutes on the second side, then slide onto a serving plate. Meanwhile heat the sauce; pour it over the *frittata,* and garnish with additional cheese, if you like, and parsley sprigs.

VARIATIONS: Add diced cooked vegetables, or small pieces of cooked chicken, turkey, ham or ground beef.

RICOTTA TORTA MARANA

TIME: 25 MINUTES
SERVINGS: 8 APPETIZER SERVINGS
CALORIES: 145 PER SERVING

> 4 *eggs*
> 1 *cup skim-milk ricotta or cottage cheese*
> 1 *cup shredded skim-milk mozzarella cheese*
> 1 *teaspoon prepared Dijon mustard*
> 2 *tablespoons snipped fresh chives*
> 3 *tablespoons chopped fresh Italian parsley*
>   *salt and pepper*
> 1 *baked whole-wheat pie shell (p. 277), 9 inches*

Preheat oven to 400°F. In a large bowl mix eggs, ricotta or cottage cheese, mozzarella cheese, mustard, chives, parsley, and salt and pepper to taste. Pour into the baked shell, and bake for 15 to 20 minutes. Serve hot or cold.

If the pie is cut into 6 pieces instead of 8, each will provide about 190 calories.

VARIATIONS: Onions, mushrooms, green peppers or asparagus, all sautéed, blanched or steamed, can be used to vary the filling.

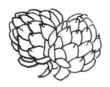

TORTINA DI CARCIOFI ALLA FIORENTINA
Baked Artichokes, Florentine Style

TIME: 20 MINUTES, EXCLUDING TIME TO COOK ARTICHOKES
SERVINGS: 6
CALORIES: 160 PER SERVING

> 4 *cooked fresh artichoke bottoms (p. 195), drained*
> 2 *tablespoons olive oil*
> 6 *eggs*
>   *salt and pepper*

When artichoke bottoms are cool enough to handle, remove all remaining leaves and the chokes. Cut bottoms into quarters or slices; there should be about 2 cups of the pieces. Heat the oil in a 4-cup flameproof baking dish that can come to the table, and lightly brown the artichokes in it. Beat the eggs until almost foamy, season with salt and pepper, and pour over the artichokes. Bake in a preheated 350°F. oven for 15 minutes, until the eggs are firm.

VARIATIONS: Lacking fresh artichokes, this dish can be made with frozen artichoke hearts. Use one 9-ounce package and cook following package directions.

For more zip, sprinkle the top of the *tortina* with grated Parmesan cheese before baking.

CHEESE AND SPINACH TORTA

TIME: 25 MINUTES
SERVINGS: 4 AS A MAIN COURSE; 8 AS A FIRST COURSE
CALORIES: 165 PER SERVING AS MAIN COURSE; 83 PER SERVING AS FIRST
                COURSE

½ *pound fresh spinach*
4 *eggs*
1 *cup skim-milk ricotta cheese*
½ *cup liquid skim milk*
3 *tablespoons grated Parmesan cheese*
1 *tablespoon prepared Dijon mustard*
1 *tablespoon Italian seasoning*
    salt and pepper
    vegetable oil for pan

Wash spinach carefully; discard damaged leaves, roots and any coarse stems.
Cook spinach in the water clinging to the leaves until just tender, about 5
minutes. Drain well and chop. There should be about ½ cup chopped.

Beat eggs lightly in a large bowl. Add ricotta and mix well. Mix in skim
milk, little by little, until you have a smooth mixture. Add spinach, Parmesan
cheese, mustard and Italian seasoning. Add salt and pepper to taste. Mix well.
Oil a 4-cup pie pan or pottery quiche dish, and spoon the filling into it;
smooth the top. Bake in a preheated 450°F. oven for 15 minutes. Serve hot
or cold as a first course with wine; or serve as a main course accompanied
with a vegetable and a green salad.

VARIATIONS: Instead of spinach, use mushrooms, onions, eggplant or zucchini. Wash, trim, or peel, according to the kind of vegetable, chop, and sauté
in about 1 tablespoon vegetable oil until just tender. After sautéing you
should have ½ cup of whichever vegetable you are using. If you like, put the
sautéed vegetable in paper towels to remove any remaining oil.

To make a slightly larger *torta,* combine spinach and one of the other
vegetables.

For a *torta* with a crust, use whole-wheat pastry (p. 277). Or make a
crumb crust with crumbled Venus Wheat Wafers, or crumbled toasted
whole-wheat bread; press the crumbs in a thin layer into the pan just before
you add the filling.

ZUCCHINI AND CHEESE TORTA

TIME: 30 MINUTES
SERVINGS: 6
CALORIES: 205 PER SERVING

½ *pound zucchini*
4 *eggs*
½ *cup diced skim-milk mozzarella cheese*
½ *cup skim-milk ricotta cheese*
¼ *cup grated Parmesan cheese*
3 *tablespoons chopped fresh Italian parsley*
2 *tablespoons chopped fresh dill*
   pinch of cayenne pepper
   salt and pepper
   pastry for 1-crust 9-inch pie (p. 277)

Preheat oven to 375°F. Wash and trim zucchini, and grate. Beat eggs lightly in a large bowl, and add cheeses, parsley, dill, cayenne, and salt and pepper to taste. Mix well. Line a 9-inch pie dish with the pastry; trim and crimp the edges. Spread the grated zucchini in the pastry and pour the cheese custard over. Bake the pie in the preheated oven for 20 minutes, or until the custard is baked in the center.

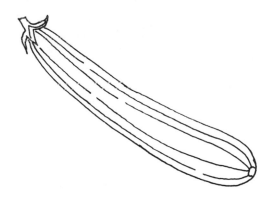

VEGETABLES

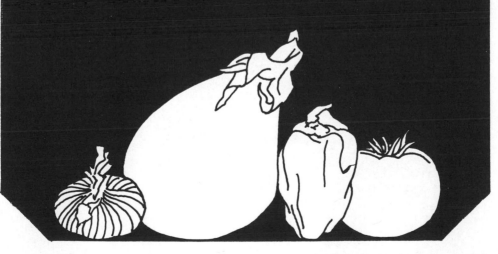

Vegetables grown in Italy have a very different taste from those found in American supermarkets. The chief reason is that they are grown differently. In Italy careful cultivation without excessive use of chemicals results in produce of superior quality. Their freshness and flavor is highlighted by the fact that they are normally served at the height of their seasons. Many Italians grow their own vegetables and herbs, but those who don't purchase vegetables fresh daily. Rather than harvesting a whole field of tomatoes, individual tomatoes are harvested as they reach perfect ripeness, leaving the rest on the vine to ripen in their turn. The perfectly grown eggplant or zucchini, or the emerald-green branches of basil—these are feasts for the eye as well as for the inner man.

When people in Italy go to the vegetable market, they are particular about selecting the right tomatoes for the pasta sauce, the perfect vegetables for the *contorni* (the accompaniment to a main dish) or first courses. The owners of vegetable markets, who may also be the growers of their gleaming produce, have pride in their merchandise that far exceeds that of a mere salesman.

Preparation has a lot to do with the taste and texture of vegetables. Almost all vegetables can be eaten raw, so overcooking them is a mistake. Vegetables should be barely cooked, still somewhat crisp and crunchy, with taste and color at the peak of perfection. It is possible to spoil them with as little as one minute too long of steaming or sautéing.

Vegetables make up a large part of the Italian diet. *Antipasti* usually include a variety of raw vegetables. Vegetables are always part of the *contorni,* and of course are the chief ingredient of salads in addition to perfect greens.

The recipes include both *contorni* (the accompaniments) and vegetable main dishes. Vegetables for first courses and salads can be found in those chapters.

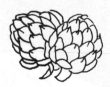

WHOLE FRESH ARTICHOKES

TIME:	25 MINUTES
SERVINGS:	4
CALORIES:	50 PER ARTICHOKE

> 4 *fresh artichokes, 8 ounces each*
> 2 *lemons, halved*
> 4 *garlic cloves, peeled*
> 1 *tablespoon salt*
> 1 *tablespoon fennel seeds, crushed in a mortar*
> 1 *large bay leaf*

Wash artichokes, break off stems, and pull off the small thin leaves at the base. With kitchen scissors snip off just the points of all the leaves. As you finish each artichoke, rub the cut portions with a lemon half, and drop artichoke and lemon into a large stainless-steel kettle holding at least 2 quarts of water. Add remaining ingredients, bring to a boil, and simmer for 15 minutes, until the base of the artichokes can easily be pierced with a stainless or silver fork. Do not overcook. Lift from the pot with tongs, drain, and serve hot or cold. Conventional service calls for vinaigrette or mayonnaise with cold artichokes, melted butter or hollandaise sauce with hot artichokes. Any of these sauces add a great many calories, and plain artichokes are delicious without further embellishment. Or try some of the low-calorie dips in Appetizers or Sauce chapters. They can serve for a first course, or as a vegetable to accompany meat or poultry.

ARTICHOKE BOTTOMS

TIME: 25 MINUTES
SERVINGS: 4
CALORIES: 35 TO 40 PER ARTICHOKE BOTTOM

An artichoke bottom is the base of a whole artichoke, with most of the leaves removed, prepared for stuffing or as an ingredient in other vegetable dishes or sauces. For stuffing use very large artichokes, ¾ to 1 pound before trimming.

Assemble the same ingredients as for cooking whole artichokes. Wash artichokes, cut off the stems level with the base, and pull off the small thin leaves at the base. With a sharp chef's knife or kitchen scissors cut off the whole leafy top, leaving a flat layer about 2 inches thick. (The large leaves that are cut off can be cooked and used for vegetable appetizers, with a dip.) With a vegetable peeler scrape off any leaf nubs from the bottom and smooth it all around. During all steps, rub cut portions with a lemon half. Drop into the pot of water, add flavoring ingredients, and simmer for 15 minutes, until the base can be pierced with a stainless or silver fork. Large bottoms may take up to 5 minutes longer, but remember that these will be cooked further, so do not let them become soft or mushy. Drain and cool.

To use for stuffing, press open the leaves to reach the choke, and scoop it out, along with all the small center leaves. Leave a rim of 2 or 3 leaves around the outside to help contain stuffing.

To use as an ingredient in other dishes, remove all leaves and choke, to have a flattened cup. These too can be stuffed, but they will hold only a small amount. Bottoms can be quartered, sliced, chopped, mashed or puréed for other recipes.

BRAISED ARTICHOKES WITH TOMATOES

TIME: 30 MINUTES, EXCLUDING TIME FOR COOKING ARTICHOKES
SERVINGS: 4
CALORIES: 65 PER SERVING

> 4 cooked artichoke bottoms (preceding recipe)
> 8 large plum tomatoes
> 1 teaspoon vegetable oil
>   juice of 1 ½ lemons
> 2 teaspoons grated lemon rind
> 4 shallots, peeled and minced
> 4 teaspoons minced fresh Italian parsley
>   salt and black pepper

Artichokes can be cooked a day ahead, and can be cooled, wrapped in moistureproof wrapping, and refrigerated. Remove leaves from artichoke bottoms and scoop out the chokes. Cut the bottoms from top to bottom into halves, to make half-moons. Plunge tomatoes into a pan of boiling water for 1 minute, then at once into a pan of cold water, and peel them. Over a strainer set in a bowl, carefully slit each tomato lengthwise, and scoop out the interior, including seeds and juice. Set the rounded side of each artichoke piece into the slit in one of the tomatoes. Using ½ teaspoon of the oil, or less, oil the bottom and sides of a 6-cup baking dish or any baking dish with a diameter of about 7 inches. Arrange the packages of artichoke and tomato around the dish in a single layer; they should just fit. Mix the tomato juice that has drained through the strainer with the lemon juice, and measure; there should be at least ½ cup. If there is less, add enough water to make up the difference. Pour the mixture over the artichokes. Mix lemon rind, shallots and parsley and scatter evenly over the top. Add a tiny pinch of salt for each little bundle and a grind of pepper (or omit salt and pepper if you prefer; salt will have been used in cooking the artichokes). With remaining oil, coat a sheet of foil, and press it, oiled side down, over the vegetables. Make a tiny hole in the center of the foil for steam to escape, and cover the baking dish. Bake in a preheated 350°F. oven for 20 minutes, or for more time at lower temperature or less time at a slightly higher temperature if you are baking something else. Lift out the foil without letting any condensed steam fall into the vegetables, and serve from the baking dish.

ARTICHOKES STUFFED WITH CHICKEN AND MUSHROOMS

TIME: 30 MINUTES, EXCLUDING TIME FOR COOKING ARTICHOKES
SERVINGS: 4
CALORIES: 230 PER SERVING

> ¾ *ounce dried mushrooms*
> 1 *cup chicken stock*
> 4 *cooked artichoke bottoms (p. 195), from 12-ounce artichokes*
> 8 *ounces poached white meat of chicken, without skin and*
>   *bones*
> 1½ *tablespoons vegetable oil*
> 6 *shallots, peeled*
> ½ *cup skim-milk ricotta cheese*
> ¼ *cup thick tomato purée*

Soak mushrooms in ¾ cup warm water for 35 minutes. Lift out and cut into pieces. Strain soaking liquid through a cloth-lined sieve and set aside. Steam mushrooms with a few tablespoons of chicken stock for 5 minutes, then turn into a bowl. Remove chokes and center leaves from artichokes, leaving a rim of leaves around the edge. Cut chicken into pieces about 1 inch square and add to mushrooms. Use a few drops of the oil to coat a baking dish, and set artichokes in it. Heat remaining oil in a skillet and chop shallots into the oil. Sauté until shallots are translucent, then add mushrooms and chicken pieces, mix well, and divide among artichokes. Mix remaining chicken stock, the ricotta, tomato purée and mushroom soaking liquid. Beat with a whisk or rotary beater and spoon over artichokes. Cover the baking dish with a tent of foil and bake in a preheated 350°F. oven for 20 minutes, until the sauce is almost bubbly. Serve as a main dish.

ASPARAGUS PONZA
Asparagus with Cheese

TIME: 15 MINUTES
SERVINGS: 4
CALORIES: 70 PER SERVING

12 *fresh asparagus*
3 *tablespoons wine vinegar*
2 *teaspoons vegetable oil*
½ *tablespoon prepared Dijon mustard*
  pepper and salt
3 *tablespoons grated Parmesan cheese*

Wash and trim asparagus and break off the tough portion of the stalks. Steam asparagus for 6 minutes. Arrange in a shallow flameproof serving dish. Mix vinegar, oil, mustard and pepper to taste; use salt sparingly, as cheese is salty. Pour over the asparagus and heat together for about 2 minutes. Sprinkle the cheese evenly on top, remove from heat, and serve at once.

ITALIAN GREEN BEANS WITH HERBS

TIME: 15 MINUTES
SERVINGS: 4
CALORIES: 60 PER SERVING

1 *pound Italian green beans*
½ *teaspoon salt*
1 *tablespoon olive oil*
4 *shallots, peeled*
2 *tablespoons minced fresh basil*
½ *teaspoon crumbled dried orégano*
2 *tablespoons lemon juice*
3 *tablespoons chopped fresh Italian parsley*

Wash beans, top and tail them, and cut diagonally into 1½-inch pieces. Put in a large saucepan, cover with cold water, add the salt, and bring to a boil. Blanch beans for 5 to 8 minutes, until barely tender; they should still be crunchy. Drain and rinse with cold water, or plunge into a pan filled with cold water. Drain again.

Heat oil in a skillet, mince shallots into oil, and sauté until they are translucent. Add basil and orégano, stir for ½ minute, then turn beans into the pan and sauté, turning until all the beans are coated with oil and herbs. Pour in lemon juice, add parsley, and keep over heat only long enough to heat everything. Serve at once.

VARIATIONS: This recipe works well for green snap beans too; they can be used whole. Wax beans are improved with the addition of the oil and herbs.

Add minced fresh dill or savory; or add minced garlic; or sprinkle with freshly ground black pepper just before serving.

If you are desperate enough to have to resort to frozen beans, this way of preparing them will greatly enhance them.

BROCCOLI ALL'OLIO
Oil-Steamed Broccoli

TIME: 12 MINUTES
SERVINGS: 4
CALORIES: 100 PER SERVING

1 ½ pounds fresh broccoli
2 tablespoons olive oil
½ garlic clove, peeled
½ teaspoon Italian seasoning
salt and pepper

Wash and trim the broccoli, peel any tough stems, and cut into small pieces of even size as much as possible. Heat the oil in a large skillet, and push the garlic through a press into the oil. Add broccoli, Italian seasoning, and salt and pepper to taste. Cover and oil-steam for 6 to 8 minutes, until broccoli is just tender—still green and a little crisp.

VARIATIONS: The same recipe can be used for spinach, asparagus or escarole.
Use shallot or onion instead of garlic.
Add sliced almonds just before serving.

EGGPLANT PARMIGIANA FRANCO

Many Italian eggplant dishes start with sautéing the slices. While it can be done, fresh eggplant absorbs a great deal of oil, and a large amount is needed for sautéing. The broiling method, which is used for other eggplant recipes in this book, gives more tender, more delicious eggplant with many fewer calories.

TIME: 30 MINUTES
SERVINGS: 6
CALORIES: 135 PER SERVING

1 *eggplant, 1½ pounds*
salt
2 *tablespoons olive oil*
½ *pound fresh plum tomatoes*
3 *shallots, peeled*
2 *tablespoons chopped fresh Italian parsley*
2 *tablespoons chopped fresh basil*
½ *cup grated Parmesan cheese*
2 *ounces skim-milk mozzarella cheese*

Wash and trim eggplant, and cut it lengthwise into thin slices. Soak the slices in cold salted water for a few minutes, then rinse in fresh water until the water is clear. Pat the slices dry. Brush a few drops of the oil on a baking sheet, and arrange the eggplant slices on it in a single layer. Slide under the broiler and broil for 5 minutes. Meantime wash and trim tomatoes, and chop; there should be 1 cup chopped.

Preheat oven to 350°F. Heat the rest of the oil in a skillet and chop the shallots into the pan. Sauté for 1 minute, then add herbs and tomatoes. Cook for 10 minutes. Spoon the sauce into a large baking dish, arrange the eggplant slices on top, and sprinkle all over with the Parmesan cheese. Cut mozzarella into thin slices, then into strips, and arrange the strips over the eggplant. Bake in the preheated oven for 15 minutes. Serve as appetizer, as main course, or as accompaniment to a main course.

VARIATIONS: Add mushrooms to the tomato sauce, or ground lean beef.

BAKED EGGPLANT CONTADINA

TIME: 30 MINUTES
SERVINGS: 6
CALORIES: 110 PER SERVING

    1 eggplant, about 1 pound
      oil
    1 pound fresh plum tomatoes
    3 shallots, peeled
    ¼ cup chopped fresh Italian parsley
    1 garlic clove, peeled
    ½ cup grated Parmesan cheese

Cut eggplant into 1-inch-thick slices, and soak slices in water to remove bitter
taste. Drain, and pat dry. Put slices on a lightly oiled pan and broil for 5
minutes on one side. Set aside. Wash and peel tomatoes, and chop; there
should be 2 cups. Pour 2 tablespoons oil into a small skillet and heat. Chop
the shallots into the pan and add the parsley. Push garlic through a press into
the mixture. Sauté until shallots become translucent. Add tomatoes and cook
until mixture is thick. Pile the vegetable mixture on the unbroiled side of the
eggplant slices, and sprinkle each one with grated cheese. Bake in a preheated 350°F. oven for 15 minutes. Use as vegetable accompaniment or
appetizer.

STUFFED EGGPLANT FRANCO

TIME: 20 MINUTES
SERVINGS: 4
CALORIES: 50 PER SERVING

    1 eggplant, about 1 pound
    1 tablespoon vegetable oil
    3 shallots, peeled
    1 garlic clove, peeled
    3 sprigs of Italian parsley
    6 fresh mushrooms, washed and trimmed
    1 tablespoon Italian seasoning
      black pepper

Wash the eggplant and remove stem and leaves, but do not peel. Cook eggplant in a large pot of water for 6 minutes, until tender. Remove from pot and heat and cool for a few minutes. Halve eggplant lengthwise and scoop out the pulp in the center without damaging the skins. Spoon the oil into a large frying pan. Chop shallots, garlic and parsley into the pan. Slice mushrooms very thin into the pan and add Italian seasoning and a dash of pepper. Sauté this mixture for 3 to 4 minutes. Add the eggplant pulp and mix well. Stuff the eggplant shells with the mixture. Bake in a preheated 350°F. oven for 10 minutes.

VARIATIONS: Top with grated Parmesan, mozzarella or ricotta cheese.
        While sautéing the filling mixture, add 1 cup tomato sauce or 1 cup cottage cheese mixed with 2 lightly beaten eggs.

STUFFED EGGPLANT FLORENCE

TIME: 25 MINUTES
SERVINGS: 4 (2 EGGPLANT HALVES EACH)
CALORIES: 160 PER SERVING

> 4 *small eggplants, about 8 ounces each*
> 4 *fresh plum tomatoes*
> 2 *anchovies*
> 2 *tablespoons olive oil*
> 1 *garlic clove, peeled*
> 6 *shallots, peeled*
> 3 *tablespoons dry red wine*
> ⅓ *teaspoon Italian seasoning*
> 6 *pink Italian olives (Gaeta), pitted and minced*
>   *salt and pepper*
> ¼ *cup chopped fresh Italian parsley*
> 3 *tablespoons grated Parmesan cheese*

Wash eggplants, remove stems and leaves, and cut them lengthwise into halves. Scoop out the pulp without damaging the shells and drop the pieces into a bowl of cold water. Drop the shells into a large pot of water, bring to a boil, and simmer for 4 minutes. Drain and set upside down. Wash tomatoes, remove hard portion near stem, and chop; there should be ½ cup. Mash the anchovies. Heat oil in a skillet and push garlic through a press into the oil. Chop shallots into the pan and add mashed anchovies. Drain eggplant pulp and dry in paper towels. Add to the skillet and sauté until shallots are translucent and eggplant lightly browned. Add wine and Italian seasoning and cook for 2 minutes. Then pour in chopped tomatoes and olives and cook until the mixture is somewhat reduced and well mixed, with everything tender. Season with salt and pepper to taste. Rub a shallow baking dish with a few drops of oil, and arrange the eggplant shells on it. Divide the filling among the shells. Mix parsley and cheese and sprinkle on the tops. Bake in a preheated 350°F. oven for 10 minutes, until eggplants are hot and cheese golden. Serve 2 halves per person, or 1 half for a first course.

EGGPLANT STUFFED WITH VEAL AND MUSHROOMS

The veal used for this dish should have been cooked by a moist method—poaching, steaming, braising—so that it is moist, with a small amount of natural gelatin coating the pieces when it is cold.

TIME: 35 MINUTES
SERVINGS: 4
CALORIES: 180 PER EGGPLANT HALF

       2 *small eggplants, about 8 ounces each*
       1 *onion, 1½ ounces*
      ¼ *pound fresh mushrooms*
      ½ *pound cooked veal, weighed after cooking and cooling*
    1½ *tablespoons vegetable oil*
       1 *tablespoon prepared Dijon mustard*
       1 *lemon*
      ¼ *cup veal stock or mushroom broth or water*
          salt
       4 *teaspoons fresh crumbs from Italian whole-wheat bread*
       4 *teaspoons grated Parmesan cheese*

Bring 1 cup of water to a boil in a large saucepan. Set a steamer basket in the pan and reduce heat so steam gently rises in the basket. Cover the saucepan. Wash eggplants, remove stem and leaves, and cut eggplants lengthwise into halves. Using a melon-ball scoop, carefully scoop out the pulp without damaging the shells. Drop the shells at once into a bowl of cold water to prevent discoloration. Without delay drop the scooped-out eggplant into the steamer and steam for 3 minutes. Dump the bits out onto a chopping board. Steam the shells, two at a time if they don't all fit, until eggplant is tender, not until it is limp. Discard the steaming liquid, as it will be bitter. Chop the eggplant bits to smaller pieces. (If eggplants are mature specimens with noticeable brown seeds, you may prefer to purée the pulp through a food mill to get rid of the seeds.) Peel and mince onion, and wash, trim, and chop mushrooms. Cut the veal into small bits.

Use ½ teaspoon oil to coat the bottom of a baking dish large enough to hold the 4 eggplant shells. Heat remaining oil in a large skillet, and sauté onion until translucent. Add the eggplant bits and veal and stir and cook until well heated. Add mushrooms and mustard, and squeeze the lemon over all. Add the stock or broth or water. Mix well and cook for 1 minute longer. Taste, and add a little salt if you like. Arrange eggplant shells in the baking dish and stuff them with the mixture. Sprinkle 1 teaspoon of crumbs and 1 teaspoon of cheese over each piece. Bake uncovered in a preheated 350°F. oven for about 20 minutes, until everything is very hot and the cheese and crumbs golden. Let eggplants wait out of the oven for 1 minute before serving, as they will be very hot.

EGGPLANT PICCANTA

TIME: 30 MINUTES
SERVINGS: 4
CALORIES: 230 PER SERVING WITH RICOTTA, 250 WITH MOZZARELLA

   3 *tablespoons vegetable oil*
   1 *cup uncooked natural brown rice*
2½ *cups water*
   salt
   1 *eggplant, 1 pound*
   2 *zucchini, 6 ounces each*
   2 *green peppers*
   3 *shallots*
   2 *garlic cloves, peeled*
  ¼ *cup chopped fresh Italian parsley*
   1 *tablespoon grated fresh gingerroot*
  ½ *teaspoon cayenne pepper*
   1 *cup skim-milk ricotta cheese, or 4 ounces (1 cup) shredded*
    skim-milk mozzarella cheese

Heat 1 tablespoon of the oil in a saucepan with a tight-fitting cover. Add rice and stir to coat every kernel with oil. Add ½ cup water, cover, and let rice cook until liquid is absorbed. Add another ½ cup water and ½ teaspoon salt, or more to your taste, and again cook until water is absorbed. Continue until the water is used and rice is cooked *al dente*. If rice is to your taste with less water, do not use it all. Turn cooked rice into an 8-cup casserole.

While rice is cooking, wash and trim eggplant; do not peel. Cut eggplant into small cubes and at once drop into a saucepan of water with a pinch of salt. Simmer for a few minutes, until tender; drain. Wash and trim zucchini, peel, and cut into small cubes. Wash and trim green peppers, discard ribs and seeds, and chop peppers. Peel and chop shallots. Heat remaining 2 tablespoons oil in a large skillet and push garlic through a press into the oil. Add chopped shallots and green peppers and diced zucchini, and sauté until shallots are translucent. Add parsley, gingerroot and cayenne, and sauté for 1 minute. Add drained eggplant cubes and cook for a few minutes, stirring constantly with a wooden spoon to blend all the ingredients. Spoon vegetable mixture on top of rice, and sprinkle the cheese over everything. Bake in a preheated 350°F. oven for 10 minutes, or until everything is as hot as you like.

VARIATIONS: If this is too "hot," use less gingerroot and cayenne.

Cook rice with chicken stock (more calories) or use ¼ cup dry Marsala or dry white wine in place of part of the water or stock.

FENNEL PARMIGIANO

TIME: 15 MINUTES
SERVINGS: 4
CALORIES: 110 PER SERVING

> 2 *large heads of fresh fennel*
> *salt*
> 1 *tablespoon vegetable oil*
> ½ *teaspoon crumbled dried orégano*
> *salt and pepper*
> ¼ *cup grated Parmesan cheese*
> ½ *cup shredded skim-milk mozzarella cheese*

Trim fennel, discard coarse outer ribs and top portions of inner ribs, and dice the hearts. Blanch in water with a little salt for 5 minutes. Drain well. Heat the oil in a large skillet, and add drained fennel, orégano, and a pinch of salt and pepper. Sauté until the fennel bits look barely gilded, then add Parmesan and mix quickly. Add mozzarella, remove from the heat, and toss until the mozzarella melts.

PEPPERS FRITTO

TIME: 20 MINUTES
SERVINGS: 4
CALORIES: 95 TO 100 PER SERVING (RED PEPPERS ARE HIGHER IN
            CALORIES)

> 6 large bell peppers, red or green, or 3 each
> 1 large onion, 3 ounces
> 2 tablespoons vegetable oil
> 1 garlic clove, peeled
>   salt and pepper

Wash and trim peppers, discard ribs and all seeds, and cut peppers into thin
slivers or chop them. Peel and chop onion. Heat the oil in a large skillet, and
push the garlic through a press into the oil. Add peppers and onion and sauté
over medium heat, stirring often, for 12 to 15 minutes, until peppers are
done to your taste. Season with salt and pepper to taste. Serve hot or cold
as vegetable accompaniment or appetizer.

STEWED BELL PEPPERS

TIME: 16 MINUTES
SERVINGS: 6
CALORIES: 100 PER SERVING

> 1 pound green peppers, about 4
> 2 pounds fresh plum tomatoes
> 2 to 3 tablespoons olive oil
> ½ cup chopped white onion
> 3 tablespoons chopped fresh Italian parsley
>   salt and pepper

Wash peppers, cut into halves, and discard stems, ribs and seeds. Cut peppers
into short thin strips. Wash and peel tomatoes, and chop. Heat 2 tablespoons
of the oil in a skillet with a cover. Sauté chopped onion and pepper strips in
oil for a few minutes. Add additional tablespoon of oil if pan becomes dry.
Add tomatoes and parsley, cover, and simmer for about 8 minutes, until
peppers are *al dente,* or as tender as you like. Season with salt and pepper
to taste.

MAMMA CELLI'S PEPPER-ZUCCHINI MISTO

TIME: 20 MINUTES
SERVINGS: 6
CALORIES: 135 PER SERVING

> 2 *large green peppers*
> 1 *large red bell pepper*
> 2 *white onions, 3 ounces each*
> 3 *zucchini, 4 ounces each*
> 1 *potato, 3 ounces*
> 3 *tablespoons vegetable oil*
> 2 *eggs*
> ¼ *cup chopped fresh Italian parsley*
>   *salt and pepper*
> 3 *tablespoons grated Parmesan cheese*

Wash peppers, cut into halves, and discard stems, ribs and seeds. Sliver or chop peppers. Peel and chop onions. Wash and trim zucchini, but do not peel. Dice zucchini. Peel potato and cut into small dice. Heat 1 tablespoon of the oil and sauté potato dice until brown. Heat the rest of the oil in a skillet and sauté chopped onions and pepper pieces until onions are translucent. Add zucchini dice and potato when it is browned. Beat eggs and parsley together and season with salt and pepper. Pour eggs into the vegetable mixture with one hand while stirring rapidly with the other. Mix everything well. Cook for a few minutes, then sprinkle with cheese and serve without delay. Use as an appetizer, or as a main course accompanied with a salad and fruit and cheese.

VARIATIONS: A good pepper-zucchini misto can be made without eggs.
Other vegetables can be substituted.

SPINACH WITH MUSHROOMS AND CHEESE

TIME: 20 MINUTES
SERVINGS: 4
CALORIES: 120 PER SERVING

  2 *pounds fresh spinach*
  ½ *pound fresh mushrooms*
  2 *tablespoons vegetable oil*
  ½ *garlic clove, peeled*
     juice of ½ lemon
     salt and pepper
  ½ *cup shredded skim-milk mozzarella cheese*

Wash spinach well and discard any damaged leaves and coarse stems. Cook in the water clinging to the leaves for 5 minutes, and drain in a colander. Chop in the colander and let it continue to drain. Wash and trim the mushrooms, and slice. Heat the oil in a large skillet and push the garlic through a press into the oil. Add mushrooms and sauté for 2 minutes. Add spinach and sauté and mix for 2 minutes longer. Sprinkle with lemon juice and add salt and pepper to taste. Add cheese and toss for 1 minute to mix. Remove from heat at once. Serve hot or cold.

VARIATION: Omit the mushrooms and serve just spinach with cheese.

SPINACH IN ORANGE SHELLS

       TIME: 10 MINUTES
    SERVINGS: 4 (2 ORANGE HALVES PER SERVING)
    CALORIES: 85 PER HALF-ORANGE

  2 *pounds fresh spinach*
  2 *tablespoons vegetable oil*
  1 *garlic clove, peeled*
  ½ *teaspoon grated nutmeg*
     salt and pepper
  4 *oranges*
  3 *tablespoons grated Parmesan cheese*

Trim spinach of any damaged leaves and coarse stems, and wash well. Cook in the water clinging to the leaves for a few minutes; drain and chop. Pour the oil into a large skillet and add the garlic clove. Heat for a few minutes, then discard garlic. Add chopped spinach and toss for a few minutes. Season with the nutmeg and salt and pepper to taste. Cut oranges into halves and remove pulp. Separate orange pulp into sections and discard membranes. Mix sections with warm spinach and divide among the 8 half-shells.

Sprinkle cheese on top and warm in a preheated 400°F. oven for a few minutes.

BROILED TOMATOES PARMESAN

TIME: 10 MINUTES
SERVINGS: 8 (1 TOMATO HALF EACH)
CALORIES: 55 PER HALF-TOMATO

> *4 firm tomatoes, about 5 ounces each*
> *½ cup grated Parmesan cheese*
> *3 tablespoons chopped fresh Italian parsley*
> *¼ teaspoon minced fresh tarragon*
> *¼ cup dry white wine*

Wash tomatoes. Remove hard portion around stem. Cut each tomato horizontally into halves, and place them, cut sides up, on a broiler pan. Mix cheese with herbs in a small bowl. Divide the cheese mixture among the tomato halves and add ½ tablespoon white wine to each half. Slide under the broiler for 5 minutes.

TOMATOES STUFFED WITH EGGPLANT

TIME: 15 MINUTES, EXCLUDING TIME FOR CHILLING PURÉE
SERVINGS: 8 (2 TOMATOES PER SERVING)
CALORIES: 21 PER TOMATO

> *16 plum tomatoes*
> *1 pound eggplant*
> *1 tablespoon olive oil*
> *1 tablespoon lemon juice*
> *1 tablespoon capers*
> *2 tablespoons minced fresh Italian parsley*
> *1 tablespoon snipped fresh chives*
> *salt*
> *16 tiny parsley sprigs or watercress sprigs*

Wash tomatoes, cut off a slice at the stem ends, and scoop out the insides without damaging the shells. (Use the scooped-out portions for tomato sauce or juice.) Drain the tomatoes upside down.

Peel eggplant, cut flesh into chunks, and steam over 1 cup of water for about 5 minutes, until tender. Turn into a food mill and purée. (This is the best method, as it removes all the seeds and any stringy portions.) There should be about 1 cup purée. Let it cool, then stir in oil, lemon juice, capers, minced parsley and snipped chives. Season with salt to taste. Spoon about 1 tablespoon into each plum tomato, top with a parsley or watercress sprig, and serve cold.

VARIATION: Omit capers and chives. Sprinkle tops of stuffed tomatoes with grated Parmesan cheese and bake in a preheated 375°F. oven for 15 minutes.

TOMATOES STUFFED WITH SPINACH AND MUSHROOMS

TIME: 15 MINUTES
SERVINGS: 4 (2 TOMATOES PER SERVING)
CALORIES: 70 PER TOMATO

     8 *medium-size tomatoes, 1 ½ pounds altogether*
     2 *pounds fresh spinach*
     2 *tablespoons vegetable oil*
     1 *garlic clove, peeled*
     2 *shallots, peeled and chopped*
     4 *large fresh mushrooms, chopped*
     ¼ *teaspoon Tabasco*
         salt
     3 *tablespoons grated Parmesan cheese*

Wash tomatoes and cut them into halves. Carefully scoop out the pulp, chop it, and let it drain in a strainer. Turn the tomato shells upside down to drain. Trim spinach of any damaged leaves and coarse stems, and wash well. Cook in the water clinging to the leaves for a few minutes; drain and chop. Heat the oil in a large skillet. Push garlic through a press into the oil, and add shallots, tomato pulp and mushrooms. Cook for a few minutes. Add chopped spinach, toss to mix, then add the Tabasco and salt to taste. Stuff the tomato shells, and sprinkle with Parmesan. Place under the broiler for a few minutes, until cheese is golden, and serve at once.

ZUCCHINI BAKED WITH CHEESE

TIME: 20 MINUTES
SERVINGS: 4
CALORIES: 115 PER SERVING

1 ½ pounds small zucchini
1 tablespoon vegetable oil
½ cup dry red wine
2 tablespoons Italian seasoning
   pepper and salt
¼ cup grated Parmesan cheese

Scrub and trim zucchini but do not peel. Cut into thin slices. Use part of the oil to coat a 4-cup baking dish, and layer the zucchini slices in the dish. Add the rest of the oil, the wine, Italian seasoning, a dash of pepper and a small sprinkle of salt (cheese is salty). Sprinkle with the cheese. Bake in a preheated 350°F. oven for 15 minutes.

ZUCCHINI STUFFED WITH ONION AND CHEESE

TIME: 25 TO 30 MINUTES
SERVINGS: 4 (2 HALVES PER SERVING)
CALORIES: 60 PER ZUCCHINI HALF

4 medium-size zucchini, about 6 ounces each
1 large onion, 4 ounces
2 tablespoons vegetable oil
1 garlic clove, peeled
2 teaspoons Italian seasoning
   salt and pepper
3 tablespoons dry red wine
¼ cup shredded skim-milk mozzarella cheese
¼ cup chopped fresh Italian parsley

Scrub and trim zucchini, but do not peel. Cut each one lengthwise into halves, and carefully scoop out the pulp without damaging the shells. Chop the scooped-out pulp and set aside. Cover the shells with cold water, bring to a boil, boil for 2 minutes, then drain and plunge into cold water. Drain the shells upside down while preparing the stuffing. Peel and chop the onion.

Heat the oil in a skillet and push the garlic through a press into the oil. Add chopped onion and zucchini pulp, Italian seasoning, and salt and pepper to taste. Sauté the mixture until zucchini is tender and everything well mixed. Add wine and cheese, and cook and mix well for a few minutes. Stuff the drained zucchini shells with the mixture. Arrange them on a lightly oiled baking sheet, and sprinkle each one with ½ tablespoon of the parsley. Bake in a preheated 400°F. oven for 15 minutes, or until done to your taste.

ZUCCHINI STUFFED WITH MEAT

TIME: 25 TO 30 MINUTES
SERVINGS: 6 (2 HALVES PER SERVING)
CALORIES: 72 PER ZUCCHINI HALF

        6 medium-size zucchini, about 6 ounces each
        6 to 8 shallots
        6 large fresh mushrooms
   1 ½ tablespoons olive oil
        1 tablespoon crushed red pepper
        ½ pound lean meat (beef, veal, chicken), ground
        3 tablespoons chopped fresh Italian parsley
        2 tablespoons dry red wine
           salt and pepper
        1 egg yolk
        2 tablespoons chopped pimientos
        1 tablespoon grated Parmesan cheese

Scrub and trim zucchini, but do not peel. Cut each one lengthwise into halves, and carefully scoop out the pulp without damaging the shells. Cover the shells with cold water, bring to a boil, boil for 2 minutes, then drain and plunge into cold water. Drain the shells upside down while preparing the stuffing. Peel and chop shallots; there should be ⅓ cup. Wash and trim mushrooms, and chop; there should be ¼ cup. Heat 1 tablespoon of the oil in a skillet and sauté zucchini pulp, shallots, mushrooms and crushed red pepper until shallots are translucent. Add ground meat, half of the parsley, and the red wine, and sauté for 2 minutes, or until the meat is cooked. Season the stuffing with salt and pepper to taste. Beat the egg yolk slightly and brush some on the inside of each zucchini boat. Fill the boats with the meat stuffing. Top each filled shell with bits of pimiento and a pinch of the cheese. Use the rest of the oil to coat a shallow baking pan. Place zucchini shells in the pan and bake in a preheated 350°F. oven for 10 minutes, or until done to your taste. Sprinkle remaining parsley on top.

VARIATIONS: Use black olives or anchovies instead of mushrooms. Use tomato sauce instead of wine.

ZUCCHINI MISTO

TIME: 15 TO 20 MINUTES
SERVINGS: 6
CALORIES: 85 PER SERVING

3 *zucchini, about 5 ounces each*
8 *fresh plum tomatoes*
2 *medium-size green peppers*
1 *large onion, 4 ounces*
4 *large fresh mushrooms*
2 *tablespoons vegetable oil*
½ *teaspoon Italian seasoning*
   black pepper
2 *tablespoons grated Parmesan cheese*
3 *tablespoons dry red wine*
   salt
1 *cup shredded lettuce, or 4 Bibb lettuce leaves*
   minced fresh Italian parsley

Scrub zucchini and trim; if they are fresh and unblemished, do not peel. Wash tomatoes and peppers; remove ribs and seeds from peppers. Peel onion. Chop all these vegetables. Wash and dry mushrooms, trim stems, and cut mushrooms into slices. Pour the oil into a large skillet and add all the chopped vegetables, the sliced mushrooms, Italian seasoning, and a dash of freshly ground black pepper. Sauté over medium heat, stirring often, until peppers become tender, about 6 minutes. Add grated cheese, stir, then add wine, and continue to cook for 5 minutes longer. Season with salt to taste. Serve warm, or chill and serve on a bed of shredded lettuce or in a perfect Bibb lettuce leaf. Sprinkle with parsley.

VARIATIONS: Serve hot; in this case you may prefer to sprinkle the cheese on top just before serving.

If you do not have good fresh tomatoes, use 1 pound canned peeled plum tomatoes. Break up the tomatoes and let them cook down with the other vegetables.

Add sliced pitted olives, only a few, or chopped red pimientos, or sliced cooked artichoke bottoms.

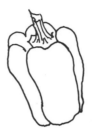

FRITTO MISTO

TIME: 15 MINUTES
SERVINGS: 6
CALORIES: 140 PER SERVING

> 1 large green pepper
> 2 potatoes, 4 ounces each
> 2 zucchini, 6 ounces each
> 1 onion, 5 ounces
> 2 tablespoons vegetable oil
> 2 garlic cloves, peeled
> ¼ teaspoon crushed red pepper
> 3 eggs, lightly beaten
> ½ teaspoon Italian seasoning
>   salt and pepper
> ⅓ cup chopped fresh Italian parsley
> 3 tablespoons grated Parmesan cheese

Wash and trim pepper, discard ribs and seeds, and dice the pepper. Peel and dice potatoes. Wash and trim zucchini, and dice. Peel and chop onion. Heat the oil in a large skillet and push the garlic through a press into the oil. Add green pepper and potatoes and sauté for a few minutes. Add zucchini, onion and crushed red pepper, and sauté and stir for 4 minutes. Add eggs, stir, then add Italian seasoning. Cook as though scrambling eggs, stirring rapidly to mix eggs and vegetables and to help eggs cook properly. Add salt and pepper to taste, and serve sprinkled with parsley and cheese.

GREEN VEGETABLE MISTO

TIME: 15 TO 20 MINUTES
SERVINGS: 8 AS A VEGETABLE; 16 AS A SAUCE
CALORIES: 65 PER SERVING; 8 PER 1 TABLESPOON

1 *pound fresh spinach*
1 ½ *pounds fresh broccoli*
2 *tablespoons olive oil*
6 *shallots, peeled*
3 *garlic cloves, peeled*
3 *tablespoons chopped fresh basil*
¼ *cup chopped fresh Italian parsley*
¼ *teaspoon grated nutmeg*
  salt and pepper
¼ *cup skim-milk ricotta cheese*
¼ *teaspoon dry mustard*

Wash spinach well and discard any damaged leaves and all stems. With scissors cut the leaves into small pieces; there should be about 2 cups. Wash and drain broccoli, and separate the flowerets. (Use stems for something else.) Chop the flowerets. Heat olive oil in a large skillet. Mince shallots into the oil, and push garlic through a press into the oil. Add spinach and broccoli and sauté, turning until all the vegetables are coated with oil. Cover the pan and steam for 5 or 6 minutes. Uncover the skillet and mix in the basil, parsley and nutmeg. Add salt and pepper to taste. Mix ricotta and dry mustard in a cup, then turn into a blender container and whirl for 1 second. Add the vegetable mixture to the container and blend for 3 or 4 seconds. Serve at room temperature, or return to the skillet and reheat to serve hot. Use as vegetable accompaniment to a main course, or serve as a sauce. MAKES ABOUT 4 CUPS.

VARIATIONS: Add 1 cup chopped fresh plum tomatoes; or add chopped asparagus, celery or zucchini.
    Use as a filling for tomatoes, or for fish rolls.

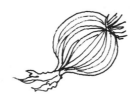

VEGETABLE CASSEROLE ALLA BRUNO

TIME: 30 MINUTES
SERVINGS: 6
CALORIES: 125 PER SERVING

1 *pound mixed vegetables (eggplant, potato, tomato, zucchini)*
2 *eggs*
1 *cup dried crumbs, made from whole-wheat Italian bread*
⅓ *cup chopped fresh Italian parsley*
¼ *cup chopped shallots*
3 *tablespoons chopped fresh basil*
⅓ *teaspoon Italian seasoning*
1 *garlic clove, peeled*
1 *tablespoon olive oil*
  salt and pepper
1 *cup diced or shredded skim-milk mozzarella cheese*

Wash and trim vegetables, peel if necessary, and cut them all into thin slices. Break the eggs into a bowl and beat until well mixed but not foamy. Stir in crumbs, parsley, shallots, basil and Italian seasoning, and push garlic through a press into the mixture; mix thoroughly. Use the oil to coat a 9-inch deep pie dish or 6-cup square or rectangular pan. Layer some of the vegetables in the oiled pan, sprinkle lightly with salt and pepper, then spoon part of the crumb mixture over. Sprinkle with part of the mozzarella. Continue with vegetables, seasoning, crumb mixture and cheese. If there is enough, make a third layer. The top layer should be cheese. Bake in a preheated 350°F. oven for 20 minutes. If you used a round pan, cut into wedges to serve. A rectangular casserole can be cut into squares.

ITALIAN VEGETABLE STEW

TIME: 20 MINUTES
SERVINGS: 6
CALORIES: 85 PER SERVING (THIS VARIES WITH THE CHOICE OF
                VEGETABLES)

    2 *pounds assorted fresh vegetables (broccoli, carrot, celery, eggplant, mushroom, onion, bell pepper, potato, tomato, zucchini)*
    1 *to 1 ½ cups water or chicken stock or veal stock*
    ⅓ *cup chopped fresh Italian parsley*
    3 *tablespoons chopped fresh basil*
    ¼ *teaspoon crumbled dried marjoram*
    2 *teaspoons olive oil*
        salt and pepper
    3 *tablespoons grated Parmesan cheese*

Wash vegetables, and trim or peel according to the kind you are using. Cut them into medium-size pieces, as nearly as possible all of the same size. Put 1 cup water or stock into a large saucepan. Use the rest of the liquid if necessary; this depends on the size and shape of the saucepan and the vegetables in the mixture—carrots and potatoes need more, celery and mushrooms less. Add first any vegetables that need longer cooking (carrots, peppers, potatoes), and cook for 2 minutes. Add the rest and simmer for 6 to 8 minutes longer, or until done to your taste. However, all vegetables taste better cooked *al dente*. Stir in all the herbs, the oil and salt and pepper to taste. Serve hot or cold, with ½ tablespoon Parmesan sprinkled over each serving. This is delicious with brown rice.

VEGETABLE TORTA CELLI

TIME: 30 MINUTES
SERVINGS: 4
CALORIES: 185 PER SERVING

    1 *pound assorted vegetables (eggplant, bell peppers, zucchini)*
    ½ *pound fresh plum tomatoes*
    6 *to 8 shallots*
    2 *tablespoons olive oil*
    2 *garlic cloves, peeled*
    ⅓ *cup chopped fresh Italian parsley*
    ½ *teaspoon crushed red pepper*
    ⅓ *teaspoon Italian seasoning*
    3 *tablespoons chopped fresh basil*
    4 *ounces skim-milk mozzarella cheese*

Wash and trim vegetables, peel if necessary, and cut them into thin slices; there should be at least 2 cups. Wash tomatoes, remove hard portion near stem, and chop; there should be 1 cup. Peel and chop shallots; there should be ⅓ cup. Use a few drops of the oil to coat a 6-cup baking dish; a 9-inch deep pie dish is a good choice. Pour the rest of the oil into a skillet. Push garlic through a press into the oil and add shallots, part of the parsley and the red pepper. Sauté until shallots are translucent, then add tomatoes, Italian seasoning, basil and remaining parsley. Cook, stirring often, until the mixture is reduced to a sauce. While it cooks, chop or shred the cheese. Layer all the ingredients in the baking dish, vegetables, tomato sauce, cheese, then another layer of each, ending with cheese. Bake in a preheated 350°F. oven for 15 minutes. Cut into wedges to serve.

VEGETABLE PURÉES

Purées can be used as a vegetable accompaniment or as a salad ingredient; they are also useful for appetizers. Use as a dip or dressing, or to stuff other vegetables. To use as a sauce, thin to the correct texture with wine or stock.

Cut the vegetable into small chunks and steam until tender. Drain if necessary. Put in a blender container with mashed hard-cooked eggs and skim-milk ricotta or cottage cheese. Add minced shallots and herbs and/or spices appropriate to the vegetable. Blend to a purée.

PROPORTIONS
> 2 cups vegetable chunks
> 1 hard-cooked egg
> 1 cup cheese
> 2 shallots, peeled and minced
> ½ to 1 teaspoon herb and/or spice

SALADS

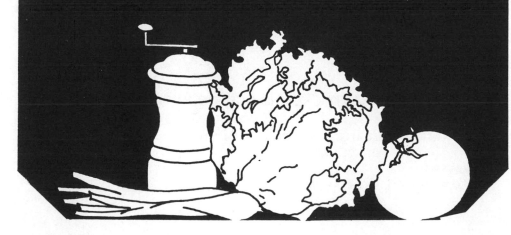

In Italy the salad follows the main course to help digest the heaviest part of the meal, and to take away the flavors of the main course, so as to prepare the taste buds for what follows—fruit and cheese, or sweets. The salad as a first course so often served in American restaurants is a device to pacify the customers while they wait for their food. What a disaster! Salad before the meal starts the digestive process before there is anything substantial to eat. Also, the taste buds are numbed for the wine or for the courses that follow. And finally, why fill up on salad and the accompanying basket of bread before the most important and exciting part of the meal arrives? The custom is said to have originated in a California restaurant that could not turn out food fast enough to please its customers. At home we urge that you follow the traditional order; the reasons for it still apply.

An Italian salad usually consists of a variety of fresh greens and raw vegetables. It is most often very simple, so that the greens can be tasted. (The greens in an Italian salad are not just a tasteless collection of leathery shreds used as a base for equally tasteless pallid tomato wedges.) Rugola, or arugula, is the star salad green in Italy; it has a great, refreshing taste. Dressings are usually light oil with vinegar or lemon juice, made for each salad just before it is served—nothing out of a bottle or package. With such a light dressing, the taste emphasis is on the greens themselves, not the dressing.

Salads are healthful, low in calories and inexpensive. If they are well prepared, they are also tasty, exciting and versatile. A variety of greens and garnishes can be used. The basic dressing can be altered by a change of herbs and seasonings. Serve salads at lunch or dinner, after the main course. One can also serve a hearty salad in place of a main course. There are many excellent greens to use; don't think only of the expensive and bland-tasting iceberg lettuce. Look for rugola, endive, escarole, romaine, watercress, fennel. Dill is an excellent herb for salads, and there are many great seasonings. All sorts of raw vegetables and fruits can be used. Also eggs, seafood, even pasta!

Salad adds necessary bulk and roughage to the diet, lots of vitamins, and satisfying good taste. Once you become a salad addict, it will become a daily requirement.

ARTICHOKE AND MUSHROOM SALAD

TIME: 10 MINUTES, EXCLUDING TIME TO COOK AND COOL
              ARTICHOKES
SERVINGS: 4
CALORIES: 90 PER SERVING

    4 *medium-size fresh artichoke bottoms, cooked (p. 195) and*
       cooled
    6 *large fresh mushrooms*
 1 ½ *tablespoons vegetable oil*
    2 *tablespoons wine vinegar*
    1 *tablespoon prepared Dijon mustard*
    1 *teaspoon Italian seasoning*
       salt and pepper
    8 *perfect lettuce leaves*

Discard any leaves and the chokes from the artichoke bottoms, and cut the bottoms into thin slices. Wash and trim mushrooms and cut into slices a little thinner than the artichoke slices. Combine the vegetables in a bowl. Mix oil, vinegar, mustard and Italian seasoning, add salt and pepper to taste, pour over the vegetables, and toss to combine well. Arrange 2 lettuce leaves on each plate and divide the salad among them.

VARIATION: Decorate with a few black olives or pimiento strips or chopped parsley, or mix any of these into the salad.

ASPARAGUS AND SCALLION SALAD

       TIME: 15 MINUTES
   SERVINGS: 4
   CALORIES: 95 PER SERVING

   10 *fresh asparagus*
    5 *scallions*
    4 *tablespoons wine vinegar*
    3 *tablespoons lemon juice*
    2 *tablespoons capers*
   ¼ *teaspoon snipped fresh tarragon*
    1 *hard-cooked egg yolk*
    1 *small head of romaine lettuce, washed and patted dry*
    2 *tablespoons vegetable oil*
       salt and pepper

Wash and trim asparagus and break off the tough portion of the stalks. Wash and trim the scallions, leaving only ½ inch of the green tops. Blanch or steam asparagus for 5 minutes, until cooked but still crunchy. At the same time steam the scallions for 4 minutes, until tender. Cool both vegetables and dice. Mix in a cup the vinegar, lemon juice, capers and tarragon. Mash the egg yolk and mix into the dressing. Break up the lettuce in a bowl and toss with the oil. Add the asparagus and scallions, pour the dressing over all, and toss. Add salt and pepper to taste if needed.

ITALIAN BEAN SALAD

TIME: 15 MINUTES
SERVINGS: 8
CALORIES: 45 PER SERVING

> 1 *pound fresh Italian green beans*
> 1 *pound fresh wax beans*
> 1 *shallot, peeled*
> 1 *garlic clove, peeled*
> 2 *tablespoons vegetable oil*
> 1 *tablespoon wine vinegar*
> 1 *teaspoon Italian seasoning*
>   *black pepper*
> 2 *tablespoons minced fresh Italian parsley*

Trim and wash green and wax beans, and cut into 1-inch pieces. Steam over 1½ cups water for 6 minutes, then plunge into cold water until beans are cooled, and drain well. Beans should still be crunchy. Put them into a salad bowl. Mince shallot into a small bowl, and put garlic through a press into the same bowl. Add oil, vinegar and Italian seasoning. Mix the dressing well, then pour over the beans and toss. Sprinkle with black pepper and the parsley.

EGGPLANT SALAD

TIME: 20 MINUTES
SERVINGS: 6
CALORIES: 85 PER SERVING

  4 *eggplants, 8 ounces each*
   salt
  3 *tablespoons olive or vegetable oil*
  2 *tablespoons red-wine vinegar*
  2 *garlic cloves, peeled*
  ½ *teaspoon crumbled dried orégano*
  3 *shallots, peeled and minced*
  ¼ *cup chopped fresh Italian parsley*

Wash eggplants, remove stems and leaves, and peel or not as you prefer. Dice the eggplant and at once drop into a pot of cold water, enough to cover all the pieces. Add 1 teaspoon salt for each quart of water. Bring to a boil, cover the pot, and simmer for 10 minutes. Drain, cool, and turn into a serving bowl. Pour oil and vinegar into a cup, and push the garlic through a press into the cup. Add orégano and mix with a fork, then pour over the eggplant and toss to mix thoroughly. Add the shallots and parsley, mix again, and serve.

   This is excellent as an appetizer. To make it spicier, add cayenne pepper to taste.

EGGPLANT AND PEPPER SALAD

  TIME: 30 MINUTES
SERVINGS: 16 (½ CUP PER SALAD SERVING), OR 32 APPETIZER SERVINGS
CALORIES: 40 PER ½ CUP

  1 *eggplant, 2 pounds*
  3 *tablespoons olive oil*
  ¼ *cup red-wine vinegar*
  2 *medium-size green peppers*
  3 *large red bell peppers*
  ⅓ *cup minced fresh Italian parsley*
  4 *plum tomatoes*
  3 *garlic cloves, peeled*
  ¼ *teaspoon cayenne pepper*
   salt

Wash eggplant, cut lengthwise into halves, and place on a baking sheet oiled with a few drops of the oil. Sprinkle 1 tablespoon of the vinegar on each cut surface, and broil for 15 minutes. At the same time trim green and red peppers, discard ribs and seeds, and cut peppers into quarters. Place skin side up on a baking sheet and broil while the eggplant is broiling, until the skin is blistered. Remove eggplant from broiler and cool enough to handle. While eggplant cools, rub off the skins of the peppers with a coarse cloth. Rinse peppers, chop into small pieces, and put into a large bowl. Discard eggplant skin and put the pulp through a food mill into the bowl with the peppers. Add parsley.

Wash tomatoes, cut out hard part around stem, and press gently to get rid of as many seeds as possible. Chop tomatoes and add to the bowl. Add remaining oil and vinegar. Push garlic through a press into the mixture. Mix with a wire whisk until everything is blended. Add as much of the cayenne as you like, and salt to taste. Serve a scoop of the purée on a lettuce leaf as salad or first course; or turn into a serving bowl, garnish with pitted ripe olives, and serve with crackers or toast squares as cocktail food; or spoon onto large tomato slices as an accompaniment to a cold poultry or meat dish.

FENNEL AND MUSHROOM SALAD

TIME: 15 MINUTES
SERVINGS: 4
CALORIES: 50 PER SERVING

2 *heads of fennel*
6 *large fresh mushrooms*
2 *shallots*
1 *small head of Boston lettuce*
2 *tablespoons wine vinegar*
1 *tablespoon olive oil*
   salt and pepper
2 *tablespoons chopped fresh Italian parsley*

Trim fennel, discard coarse outer ribs and top portions of inner ribs, and chop the hearts into large pieces. Wash and trim mushrooms and cut into thin slices. Peel and chop shallots. Shred lettuce and divide among 4 plates, or arrange in a salad bowl. Toss fennel and mushrooms together and place on the lettuce bed. Sprinkle shallots on top. Mix vinegar and oil and add salt and pepper to taste. Spoon over the vegetables, and sprinkle all with parsley.

FENNEL AND RUGOLA SALAD

TIME: 6 MINUTES
SERVINGS: 4
CALORIES: 50 PER SERVING, WITHOUT APPLE

    1 *large head of fennel*
    1 *large red apple (optional)*
    2 *small bunches of rugola*
    1 *tablespoon vegetable oil*
    2 *tablespoons snipped fresh dill*
    ½ *tablespoon Italian seasoning*
    ½ *teaspoon white pepper*
       juice of ½ lemon

Remove coarse outer ribs and top portion of fennel, leaving only the crisp heart. With a sharp knife cut this into thin strips. Cut the unpeeled apple into thin slivers. Wash and trim the rugola and dry in a towel. Put rugola, fennel and apple in a large bowl and toss gently to mix. Add the oil and toss again. Mix herbs, pepper and lemon juice and add to salad. Toss well and chill.

VARIATIONS: Add thin slices of fresh mushrooms to the fennel and apple.
    Add ½ teaspoon prepared Dijon mustard to the dressing.

FENNEL AND ZUCCHINI SALAD

TIME: 5 MINUTES
SERVINGS: 4
CALORIES: 55 PER SERVING

    1 *large head of fennel*
    1 *small zucchini, about 4 ounces*
    4 *small tomatoes*
    ¼ *cup snipped fresh dill*
    1 *tablespoon Italian seasoning*
       salt and pepper
       few drops of sesame or vegetable oil
    ¼ *cup Vinaigrette Dressing (p. 254)*

Remove coarse outer ribs and top portion of fennel, leaving only the crisp heart. Cut into small dice. Peel and dice the zucchini. Dice the tomatoes. Put vegetables in a large bowl. Add dill and Italian seasoning, and salt and pepper to taste. Coat the salad with a few drops of sesame or vegetable oil. Prepare the dressing separately and pour over the salad. Toss to mix, and serve.

VARIATIONS: Use watercress instead of zucchini, or lettuce, endive or rugola.
    Add crushed peeled garlic or minced shallots.
    Instead of tomatoes, use 2 small pimientos, well drained and diced.

MUSHROOM SALAD

TIME: 5 MINUTES
SERVINGS: 2
CALORIES: 87 PER SERVING

    6 *large fresh mushrooms*
    1 *tablespoon olive oil*
    1 *tablespoon white-wine vinegar*
    1 *tablespoon prepared Dijon mustard*
       garlic salt
       black pepper
    2 *perfect Bibb lettuce leaves*
    2 *teaspoons snipped fresh chives*

For this use only perfect, unblemished white mushrooms. Wash mushrooms; do not peel, but cut off the stem ends. Cut through cap and stem to make very thin slices. Mix the dressing—oil, vinegar and mustard—and season with garlic salt and black pepper to your taste. Gently turn the raw mushroom slices in the dressing until well coated. Spoon onto the lettuce leaves on 2 plates, and sprinkle the chives on top.

VARIATIONS: Instead of serving the salad in a lettuce cup, use more lettuce and cut into shreds for a base.
    While this is good plain, it can be augmented with chopped onion, sliced black olives, chopped pimientos, sliced or chopped celery, chopped parsley, or slivers of cooked artichoke bottom. With any of these additions, the salad will make more servings.
    Instead of vinegar, use lemon juice. Instead of mustard, use 1 tablespoon drained capers.

STELLA'S INSALATA

TIME: 25 MINUTES
SERVINGS: 4
CALORIES: 100 PER SERVING

4 large green peppers
1 pound fresh plum tomatoes
2 tablespoons olive oil
2 garlic cloves, peeled
¼ cup chopped fresh Italian parsley
¼ teaspoon Italian seasoning
    salt and pepper

Wash green peppers, cut into halves, and discard ribs and all seeds. Place pepper halves, skin side toward the heat, on a baking sheet, and broil for 10 minutes. When peppers are cool enough to handle, rub off the skins with a coarse cloth. Cut peppers into small dice. While peppers are broiling, dip tomatoes into boiling water for a few minutes, then into cold water. Pull off skins. Cut tomatoes into small dice. Heat the oil in a large skillet and push the garlic through a press into the oil. Add tomato dice and part of the parsley and Italian seasoning, and sauté for 5 minutes. Add pepper dice and remaining parsley and Italian seasoning. Cover the skillet and cook for 5 minutes. Taste, and add salt and pepper as needed. Serve hot as a vegetable or cold as a salad.

VARIATION: Do not sauté vegetables. Combine tomato and pepper dice, parsley and Italian seasoning, and toss with oil and garlic in a bowl. Season to taste and serve cold.

POTATO SALAD NESTORIA

TIME: 10 MINUTES, EXCLUDING TIME TO BOIL POTATOES
SERVINGS: 4
CALORIES: 65 PER SERVING

2 potatoes, 4 ounces each, boiled
1 tablespoon olive oil
¼ cup chopped fresh Italian parsley
    salt and freshly ground pepper

Drain and cool potatoes, and peel. Cut them into thin wedges and arrange the wedges on a small serving platter. Pour the oil over the potatoes and sprinkle them with parsley and salt and pepper to taste. Serve at room temperature or cool.

WATERCRESS AND APPLE SALAD

TIME: 10 MINUTES
SERVINGS: 4
CALORIES: 25 PER SERVING

    1 large bunch of watercress
    1 large red-skinned apple
      juice of 1 lemon

Wash watercress thoroughly and roll in a towel to dry. Pull all the leaves off the watercress and discard the stems. Wash apple, but do not peel; remove stem and blossom ends, and cut into quarters. Remove the core portion and slice each quarter into thin slices. Mix in a bowl with the watercress leaves and sprinkle lemon juice over all.

WATERCRESS AND CUCUMBER SALAD

TIME: 10 MINUTES
SERVINGS: 4
CALORIES: 80 PER SERVING

    1 large bunch of watercress
    2 medium-size young cucumbers
    3 tomatoes
    2 tablespoons wine vinegar
    1 tablespoon vegetable oil
    1 tablespoon prepared Dijon mustard
      salt and pepper

Wash watercress thoroughly and roll in a towel to dry. Pull all the leaves off the watercress and discard the stems. Scrub cucumbers, but do not peel. Cut off the ends, then with a fork score the peel from end to end (to give a striped or scalloped edge when cut). Cut scored cucumbers into very thin slices. Wash tomatoes and remove hard portion near the stem. Cut each tomato into quarters, then halve the quarters across. Mix watercress, cucumber slices and tomato pieces in a large serving bowl. Mix the vinegar, oil and mustard in a cup, adding salt and pepper to taste, and toss with the salad just enough to mix well. If you do not plan to serve the salad at once, keep it chilled and add the dressing just before serving.

WATERCRESS AND FENNEL SALAD

TIME: 15 MINUTES, EXCLUDING TIME FOR CHILLING
SERVINGS: 6
CALORIES: 20 PER SERVING

1 large bunch of watercress
2 large heads of fennel
6 very small tomatoes
2 tablespoons minced fresh mint
2 shallots, peeled and minced
salt and pepper

Wash watercress, discard stems, and put the leaves in a large bowl. Wash fennel, discard coarse outer ribs, and dice the hearts. Wash and slice tomatoes. Add both to watercress. Add mint, shallots, and salt and pepper to taste. Chill. Serve with Lemon Dressing or Vinaigrette Dressing (see Index).

ZUCCHINI SALAD DI CARLO

TIME: 10 MINUTES, EXCLUDING TIME TO COOL THE VEGETABLES
SERVINGS: 4
CALORIES: 75 PER SERVING

2 medium-size zucchini, about 5 ounces each, not waxed
3 tomatoes, about 5 ounces each
1 onion, 1 ounce
1 tablespoon vegetable oil
1 teaspoon Italian seasoning
salt and pepper
1 cup shredded lettuce
1 teaspoon snipped fresh chives

Scrub and trim zucchini but do not peel. Cut into very thin slices. Wash tomatoes and remove hard portion near stem. Cut into small dice. Peel and chop onion. Heat the oil in a skillet and add all the vegetables and the Italian seasoning. Sauté, stirring often, for 5 minutes. Season with salt and pepper to taste, and let the mixture cool. Serve over a bed of shredded lettuce, and sprinkle with the chives.

ZUCCHINI AND BROCCOLI SALAD

TIME: 6 MINUTES
SERVINGS: 6
CALORIES: 125 PER SERVING

> 1 pound fresh broccoli
> 4 zucchini, about 1 pound, not waxed
> 4 red pimientos, drained
> 3 scallions, trimmed
> 1 bunch of watercress, washed and dried
> 3 tablespoons vegetable oil
> 5 tablespoons wine vinegar
> 2 teaspoons minced fresh tarragon
> 3 tablespoons minced fresh dill
>   salt and pepper
> 2 medium-size red apples, unpeeled
>   juice of ½ lemon

Wash and drain broccoli. Break off broccoli flowerets and slice into a large bowl. (Use the rest of broccoli for something else.) Scrub zucchini, and score lengthwise from end to end with tines of a fork. Cut zucchini into thin crosswise slices. Add to broccoli. Slice pimientos and scallions into the bowl. Break watercress sprigs from stems and add sprigs to bowl. (Save stems for stock or soup.) In a cup mix the oil, vinegar, tarragon and dill to make a dressing. Add salt and pepper to taste. At serving time toss dressing with vegetables. Cut unpeeled apples into very thin slices and dip them into lemon juice to prevent discoloration. Arrange apple slices around the top of the salad. Great for buffets!

VARIATIONS: If you prefer, blanch or steam the broccoli and zucchini for a few minutes, then refresh in cold water and drain before starting to make the salad. This method requires more time, about 15 minutes.

Instead of apples, use other fruits or cheese or olives as a garnish.
Add sliced fresh mushrooms or tiny whole cherry tomatoes.
Instead of scallions, use 3 chopped shallots.
Add 1 tablespoon prepared Dijon mustard to the dressing.

MOLDED TOMATO SALAD WITH ZUCCHINI

TIME: 20 MINUTES, EXCLUDING TIME FOR CHILLING
SERVINGS: 6
CALORIES: 40 PER SERVING

2 envelopes (7 grams each) unflavored gelatin
½ cup cold water
2 cups canned peeled plum tomatoes
2 garlic cloves, peeled
1 onion, 3 ounces, peeled
2 cloves
1 teaspoon sugar
½ teaspoon Italian seasoning
2 zucchini, 4 ounces each
2 tablespoons capers
  oil for mold

Sprinkle gelatin over the cold water in a bowl and set aside to soften. Pour
tomatoes into a saucepan and push garlic through a press into the pan. Cut
onion into 4 chunks and stick the cloves into two of them. Add sugar and
Italian seasoning. Simmer the tomatoes for 12 minutes, then push through
a food mill into a clean saucepan. With a spatula scrape the gelatin into
strained tomatoes and stir over low heat until gelatin is completely dissolved.
While tomatoes are simmering, wash and trim zucchini, scrape them, and
chop or shred them. Add zucchini shreds and capers to tomato mixture, and
let it cool. When cool enough to refrigerate, chill until syrupy, stirring occasionally. Oil a 3-cup mold, and pour or spoon the aspic into it. Chill for 2
hours, until firm. Unmold to serve.

A star-shaped mold is attractive for this. The recipe can be multiplied
and molded in a larger mold or flat pan for buffet serving. The mold can be
decorated before it is filled; arrange fennel leaves and zucchini cutouts on
the bottom of the mold and attach them with clear aspic before filling the
mold. The decorations will be on top when aspic is unmolded.

VEGETABLE SALAD ISCHIA

TIME: 20 MINUTES, EXCLUDING TIME FOR CHILLING
SERVINGS: 8
CALORIES: 90 PER SERVING

 2 *white potatoes, 3 ounces each*
1 ½ *pounds fresh broccoli*
 ¾ *pound fresh green beans*
 4 *zucchini, 4 ounces each*
 ½ *pound fresh plum tomatoes*
 ½ *cup chopped celery*
 ½ *cup chopped scallions*
 ¼ *cup chopped fresh Italian parsley*
 1 *tablespoon minced fresh basil*
 3 *tablespoons red-wine vinegar*
 3 *tablespoons lemon juice*
 2 *tablespoons vegetable oil*
 1 *tablespoon prepared Dijon mustard*
    salt and pepper

Scrub potatoes, cover with cold water, cover the pan, and boil for 15 minutes, until tender. Drain and cool. While potatoes cook, blanch broccoli and green beans: Trim broccoli to flowerets (use stem portions for another recipe). Wash beans, top and tail them, and cut into 1-inch slices. In separate pans cover broccoli and beans with cold water, bring to a boil, and simmer for 5 minutes. Drain and cool. Scrub and trim zucchini and cut into thin round slices. Wash tomatoes, cut out hard portion near stem, and dice tomatoes. Peel cooked potatoes and cut into thin slices. Put all these vegetables in a large bowl with celery, scallions and herbs. Mix remaining ingredients for a dressing, with salt and pepper to taste, and pour over vegetables. Toss gently to mix, and chill until time to serve.

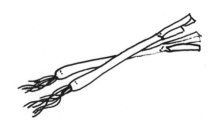

MIXED SQUASH SALAD

TIME: 15 MINUTES
SERVINGS: 4
CALORIES: 90 PER SERVING

3 zucchini, 8 ounces each
2 yellow summer squash, 8 ounces each
1 eggplant, 10 ounces
8 to 12 shallots
1 tablespoon vegetable or olive oil
1 garlic clove, peeled
  juice of 1 lemon
¼ cup minced fresh Italian parsley
2 tablespoons white-wine vinegar
1 tablespoon prepared Dijon mustard
2 tablespoons minced fresh dill
  salt and pepper

Wash and trim zucchini, yellow squash and eggplant. Peel or not as you prefer, but it is not necessary. Slice the vegetables; if they are fat the slices can be halved or quartered. Steam squash and eggplant slices for 4 to 6 minutes, until tender; the freshness of the vegetables will determine the exact time. If your vegetable steamer is small, do the steaming in batches. Let the vegetables cool. Peel and mince shallots; there should be ⅓ cup.

Spoon oil into a small bowl and push garlic through a press into the oil. Add lemon juice, parsley and shallots, and mix well. Put cooled vegetables in a large salad bowl and toss with the dressing. Separately mix vinegar, mustard and dill, pour into salad, and toss again. Season salad with salt and pepper to taste.

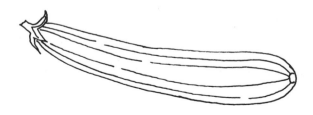

INSALATA DAVID

TIME: 25 TO 30 MINUTES
SERVINGS: 4
CALORIES: 235 PER SERVING

½ *pound fresh green beans*
1 *potato, 4 ounces*
2 *heads of romaine lettuce*
1 *large green pepper*
2 *tomatoes, 4 ounces each*
2 *pimientos*
2 *hard-cooked eggs*
2 *anchovy fillets, drained*
2 *shallots*
6 *pitted black olives*
2 *tablespoons olive oil*
2 *tablespoons red-wine vinegar*
1 *teaspoon dry mustard*
2 *tablespoons capers*
⅓ *cup chopped fresh Italian parsley*
¼ *teaspoon Italian seasoning*
   salt and black pepper
¾ *cup diced cooked tuna, or cooked chicken, turkey, or ham*

Wash beans, top and tail them, and cover with cold water. Bring to a boil and cook for 3 minutes. Drain, rinse with cold water, and drain again. Cut the beans into 1-inch pieces. Scrub potato and cook in simmering water for 15 minutes, or until tender. Drain, cool quickly, and peel. Cut into thin slices, then into sticks. Wash lettuce, drain, and break into small pieces. Roll in a towel to dry. Wash and trim green pepper, discard ribs and seeds, and chop pepper. Wash tomatoes, discard hard portion near stem, and chop. Rinse seeds from pimientos and chop. Shell and chop eggs. Mince anchovy fillets, peel and mince shallots, and chop olives.

In a small bowl mix oil, vinegar and mustard until mustard is dissolved. Stir in the capers, half of the parsley, the Italian seasoning, minced anchovies and minced shallots. Add salt and pepper to taste. Place lettuce in a bowl and spoon a little of the dressing over it. Toss to mix well, then arrange lettuce on a large platter. Toss the other ingredients, one at a time, with a small amount of dressing, and arrange them on the lettuce in a pattern—beans, potato sticks, pepper dice, tomato dice, chopped pimientos, chopped eggs and the tuna or meat. Sprinkle any remaining dressing over all, and garnish with remaining parsley and chopped olives.

SAUCES
AND DRESSINGS

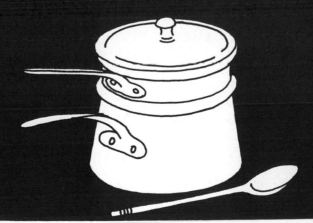

Most dishes in this book have their sauces built in—made in the same skillet or saucepan as the main ingredients are being cooked. This is typical of Italian home cooking, which does not emphasize the sauce at the expense of the fish or meat, but uses light sauces that complement the basic ingredient. Historically heavy and spicy sauces were used (in the cuisines of other countries, though seldom in Italy) to disguise the taste of spoiled foods. Our emphasis is on the freshness of all the ingredients. Fresh fish should have only a delicate sauce so that it's possible to savor the good taste of the fish; it is a waste to overpower such a delicacy. These principles apply to all the foods; no sauce should camouflage the basic tastes.

Since most of the recipes are simple, you can easily use the sauce of a fish preparation for chicken or veal, and chicken or veal sauces can be adapted for fish. In the same way the uncooked tomato sauce for pasta on page 70 can be used for *risotto,* for a *frittata,* with other vegetables, and certainly with meats. Most of the pasta sauces can be adapted for *risotto* and *frittata.*

This chapter has recipes for some of the classic light sauces of Italy, but also adaptations and original creations. The tastes come from herbs and various liquids—wine, stock, tomatoes, in a few cases milk. No sauces require lengthy cooking times.

Use your imagination in changing the ingredients of these sauces and making new combinations. What you have in your kitchen, what fits the occasion, your mood as you plan—all these factors should determine your selection. The only thing you must remember is that the best sauce is made of the finest, freshest ingredients; the best requires the best.

RICOTTA SAUCE

TIME: 5 MINUTES
SERVINGS: 6 (4 TABLESPOONS EACH)
CALORIES: 56 PER 4 TABLESPOONS

   1 cup skim-milk ricotta cheese
   ¼ cup liquid skim milk
   2 sprigs of Italian parsley, snipped
   1 teaspoon Italian seasoning
   ¼ cup grated Parmesan cheese
      black pepper

Put ricotta, skim milk, parsley and Italian seasoning in a small saucepan over medium heat. Stir often with a wooden spoon. When well mixed and hot, stir in Parmesan cheese and pepper to taste. Continue to heat and stir until Parmesan is melted. Serve at once. Makes 1½ cups.

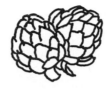

GUIDO'S ARTICHOKE SAUCE
For Pasta, Fish, Chicken, Veal

TIME: 10 MINUTES, EXCLUDING TIME TO COOK ARTICHOKES
SERVINGS: 6 (4 TABLESPOONS PER SERVING)
CALORIES: 70 PER 4 TABLESPOONS

3 large cooked fresh artichoke bottoms (see p. 195)
2 tablespoons olive oil
⅓ cup chopped shallots (6 to 8 shallots)
⅓ teaspoon grated nutmeg
¼ cup dry white wine
salt and pepper

Remove all leaves and the chokes from cooked artichoke bottoms. Chop them, then mash them; there should be about 1 cup mashed artichoke. Heat the oil in a small saucepan and sauté shallots in it until they are translucent and tender. Add mashed artichoke, nutmeg and wine, and cook and stir until the sauce is smooth like a paste, but not dry. Add a little bit more wine if sauce becomes too dry. Season to taste. Serve hot or cold. Good with fettuccine or ziti or other thicker types of pasta.

VARIATIONS: For a creamy texture, use a small amount of milk, cream or whipped skim-milk ricotta cheese.
    For a light texture, add a few tablespoons of tomato sauce.

EGGPLANT SAUCE BEPPE

TIME: 20 MINUTES
SERVINGS: 16 (5 TABLESPOONS EACH)
CALORIES: 25 PER 5 TABLESPOONS

3 *green peppers, washed and trimmed*
3 *shallots, peeled*
3 *sprigs of Italian parsley*
6 *large fresh firm tomatoes*
2 *medium-size eggplants, about 1 pound each*
1 *tablespoon vegetable oil*
1 *garlic clove, peeled*
1 *tablespoon Italian seasoning*
  black pepper
  salt

Dice the green peppers and shallots. With kitchen scissors snip parsley to bits, including the stems. Peel the tomatoes and trim stem ends. Chop tomatoes to small pieces. Peel the eggplants last (lest they discolor). Heat the oil in a large frying pan over high heat and dice the peeled eggplant into the oil. Add diced green peppers and shallots, and push the garlic through a press into the mixture. Mix well. Reduce heat to medium and cook for 3 minutes. Add snipped parsley, chopped tomatoes, Italian seasoning, and black pepper to taste. Continue to cook for 8 to 10 minutes. Stir often with a wooden spoon to mix the ingredients and to help everything cook faster. The mixture will be well reduced and ready to use at the end of 10 minutes, but you can cook it a little longer if you prefer a softer texture. Add salt to taste. Makes 5 cups.

VARIATIONS: Instead of eggplant, use the same weight of zucchini. If fresh from the garden, don't peel. If they are market vegetables with tougher skins, scrape with a vegetable peeler, taking off the thinnest possible layer of skin.

With either eggplant or zucchini, add chopped or sliced olives.

Instead of green peppers, use hot peppers, according to your taste.

If fresh tomatoes are not available, use 2 cups canned peeled plum tomatoes.

Omit tomatoes and instead use 2 cups dry red wine.

Instead of peeling eggplants, leave the purple skin on the pieces. It will add quite a different taste and color to the finished sauce.

For a smooth sauce, purée in a blender or through a food mill. The food mill will remove tomato and eggplant seeds, an important difference for an ulcer patient. Reheat the sauce to serve.

CREAMY FENNEL SAUCE
For Fish, Pasta, Veal, Chicken

TIME: 17 MINUTES
SERVINGS: 12 (4 TABLESPOONS EACH)
CALORIES: 43 PER 4 TABLESPOONS

1 *large head of fennel*
4 *shallots*
1 *garlic clove*
2 *sprigs of Italian parsley*
3 *tablespoons vegetable oil*
1 *tablespoon chopped fresh basil*
2 *tablespoons Italian seasoning*
½ *cup skim-milk ricotta cheese*
¼ *cup liquid skim milk*
sprinkle of cayenne pepper
salt and white pepper

Remove coarse outer ribs and top portion of fennel, leaving only the crisp heart. Cut into very fine dice. Cover fennel with cold water, bring quickly to a boil, and boil for 1 minute. Drain and refresh with cold water. Peel shallots and garlic, and wash and dry parsley sprigs.

Pour the oil into a large frying pan. As the oil heats, cut the shallots, garlic and parsley and drop into the oil. Add diced fennel, basil and Italian seasoning and cook for 10 minutes, turning over in the pan now and then. Fennel gets soft, yet has a "bite."

Put ricotta, skim milk and a sprinkle of cayenne in a small saucepan and heat for a few minutes, until the texture is smooth. Add more skim milk if necessary. Add cheese mixture to fennel mixture and stir over low heat until smooth, about 5 minutes. Add salt and white pepper to taste. Taste, and add more cayenne or herbs if you like. MAKES ABOUT 3 CUPS.

VARIATIONS: Use as a cold sauce, with chopped dill in place of the other herbs, or as an additional herb.

Add chopped mushrooms; sauté these with the shallots before adding the other ingredients.

CAPER SAUCE PASQUALE
For Pasta and Fish

TIME: 10 MINUTES
SERVINGS: 8 (4 TABLESPOONS EACH)
CALORIES: 50 PER 4 TABLESPOONS

½ pound fresh plum tomatoes
2 tablespoons vegetable oil
4 shallots, peeled
1 white onion, 5 ounces, peeled
3 tablespoons chopped fresh Italian parsley
2 tablespoons vinegar
¼ cup tomato paste
¼ cup capers
salt and pepper

Wash and peel tomatoes and chop. There should be about 1 cup. Heat oil in a skillet and chop shallots and onion into the oil. Add half of the parsley and sauté until onion is translucent. Add vinegar and cook for a minute, then add chopped tomatoes and tomato paste and cook for 5 minutes. Add capers and seasoning to taste and cook for 2 or 3 minutes more. Stir in remaining parsley. MAKES ABOUT 2 CUPS.

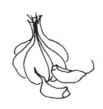

CAPER, OLIVE AND TOMATO SAUCE
For Pasta, Fish, Veal

TIME: 16 MINUTES
SERVINGS: 12 (4 TABLESPOONS EACH)
CALORIES: 40 PER 4 TABLESPOONS

> 2 tablespoons vegetable oil
> 1 garlic clove, peeled
> 3 shallots, peeled
> 1 pound fresh tomatoes
> 6 ounces tomato paste
> ¼ cup chopped fresh Italian parsley
> ½ cup capers
> 6 pink Italian olives (Gaeta) or hard green olives, chopped
>   salt and pepper

Heat the oil in a large skillet. Purée the garlic through a press into the oil, and mince the shallots into the pan. Sauté until shallots are translucent. Wash the tomatoes and remove hard portions around the stems. Dice tomatoes into the skillet and add tomato paste and parsley. Cook for 5 minutes. Add capers and olives and cook for another 5 minutes. Season with salt and pepper to taste. MAKES ABOUT 3 CUPS.

VARIATIONS: Add seafood to the sauce, or diced mushrooms.

SALSA ALLA ENRICO
Tomatoes, Olives, Anchovies—for Pasta

TIME: 20 MINUTES
SERVINGS: 12 (4 TABLESPOONS EACH)
CALORIES: 58 PER 4 TABLESPOONS

> 1 pound fresh plum tomatoes
> 3 tablespoons olive oil
> 3 salted anchovy fillets
> 2 garlic cloves, peeled
> 6 ounces tomato paste
> 5 sprigs of Italian parsley, snipped
> 5 fresh basil leaves, snipped
> 10 pitted purple Italian olives
> 2 tablespoons capers
>   salt and black pepper

Peel the tomatoes and remove hard portion at stem end. Dice the tomatoes. Pour the oil into a skillet and add anchovies. Push garlic through a press into the pan, and sauté for a few minutes. Add diced tomatoes, tomato paste, parsley and basil. Cook over medium heat for 10 minutes. Chop the olives and add with the capers to the sauce. Continue cooking for 5 minutes longer. Season with salt and black pepper to taste. MAKES ABOUT 3 CUPS.

ENRICO'S PESTO
For Pasta, Risotto, Fish, Eggs

For the perfect taste of this simple sauce with so few ingredients, use only the finest quality for each ingredient. Use no garlic or salt or pepper.

TIME: 5 MINUTES
SERVINGS: 5 OR 6 (3 TABLESPOONS EACH)
CALORIES: 50 PER TABLESPOON

2 cups large fresh basil leaves without stems
½ cup grated pecorino cheese
¼ cup olive oil

Wash basil leaves thoroughly, and dry. Put in a blender container with the cheese and oil, and blend for 5 seconds, until smooth and creamy. Stop the machine and stir with a spoon at intervals. Refrigerate to serve cold, or warm for a few minutes to serve hot. Cover with a thin film of oil, or press a sheet of plastic film tightly over the surface if you store *pesto*, lest it turn black. MAKES ABOUT 1 CUP.

VARIATIONS: Add more cheese, less oil. If pecorino cheese is not available, use Parmesan.

AL'S PESTO WITH SPINACH

It isn't easy to find fresh basil during the winter and early spring. Frozen basil can be used, but it's hardly necessary to say that dried basil is useless for *pesto*. (You can raise basil indoors but it isn't easy.) This recipe was devised for the seasons when basil is scarce, but you will need some or it isn't *pesto*.

TIME: 10 MINUTES
SERVINGS: ABOUT 10 (¼ CUP EACH)
CALORIES: 110 PER ¼ CUP

> 3 cups fresh spinach leaves without stems
> 1 cup chopped fresh Italian parsley
> ½ cup fresh basil leaves without stems
> 2 garlic cloves, peeled
> ¼ cup olive oil
> ½ cup grated Parmesan cheese
> ⅓ cup grated pecorino cheese
> 6 tablespoons hot water

Put spinach, parsley and basil in a blender container. Push garlic through a press into the mixture and add oil and cheeses. Process until the sauce is smooth. Mix in the hot water; use water from cooking pasta if you are preparing this to serve with pasta. However, this sauce has many other uses; it can be added to *risotto,* vegetables, soups. MAKES ABOUT 2½ CUPS.

SALSA VERDE
Green Sauce for Seafood, Boiled Meats, Eggs, Pasta, Risotto

TIME: 10 MINUTES, EXCLUDING CHILLING
SERVINGS: 10 (3 TABLESPOONS EACH)
CALORIES: 50 PER 3 TABLESPOONS

> ½ cup chopped fresh Italian parsley
> ¼ cup chopped shallots
> 3 tablespoons chopped fresh basil
> 3 tablespoons snipped fresh chives
> 2 garlic cloves, peeled and crushed
> 1 teaspoon chopped fresh tarragon
> 3 tablespoons olive oil
> ¼ cup red-wine vinegar
>   juice of ½ lemon
> 1½ tablespoons prepared Dijon mustard
> 1 hard-cooked egg, mashed
>   salt and pepper

In a large bowl combine all the ingredients but the egg and seasoning. Mix well. Put in a blender container and whirl for a few seconds. (Do not over-blend, as the sauce needs texture.) Add the egg and blend for another second. Add salt and pepper to taste. Chill, or serve at room temperature. MAKES ABOUT 1¾ CUPS.

VARIATION: Heat this sauce for a few minutes, and pour over pasta or *risotto,* or over a *frittata.*

NINO'S SALSA VERDE

TIME: 10 MINUTES
SERVINGS: ABOUT 6 (¼ CUP EACH)
CALORIES: 40 PER ¼ CUP

    2 *cups chopped fresh Italian parsley*
    ½ *cup fresh basil leaves without stems*
    8 *to 10 shallots*
    1 *garlic clove, peeled*
    1 *tablespoon olive oil*

Put parsley and basil in a blender container. Peel and mince shallots; there should be ½ cup. Add shallots to green herbs, and push garlic through a press into the mixture. Add oil and whirl for a few seconds, until smooth. Serve with vermicelli or other thin pasta. This can be a hot or cold sauce. MAKES ABOUT 1½ CUPS.

MARINARA SAUCE ALLA ROSA
For Pasta, Fish, Chicken, Veal

TIME: 10 MINUTES
SERVINGS: 4 (¼ CUP EACH)
CALORIES: 80 PER ¼ CUP

    ½ *pound fresh plum tomatoes*
    2 *tablespoons olive oil*
    2 *garlic cloves, peeled*
    ⅓ *cup chopped fresh Italian parsley*
    1 *large bay leaf*
       salt and pepper

Wash and peel tomatoes, and chop. There should be 1 cup. Heat oil in a skillet, and push garlic through a press into the oil. Add half of the parsley and sauté for a few minutes. Add tomatoes, bay leaf and salt and pepper to taste. Cook over medium heat, stirring well with a wooden spoon, for 3 minutes. Remove bay leaf, add remaining parsley, and cook for 2 minutes longer. MAKES ABOUT 1 CUP.

TOMATO SAUCE PIEDMONT STYLE
For Pasta, Beef, Chicken

TIME: 25 MINUTES
SERVINGS: 6 (5 TABLESPOONS EACH)
CALORIES: 80 PER 5 TABLESPOONS

    7 ripe plum tomatoes
    1 yellow onion, 4 ounces
    3 garlic cloves
    1 carrot
    3 tablespoons olive oil
    ½ teaspoon crushed red pepper
    1 teaspoon red-wine vinegar
    ¼ cup chopped fresh Italian parsley
       salt and pepper

Wash tomatoes and cut out hard portion around stem. Peel onion and garlic cloves, and scrape carrot. Pour oil into a skillet. Dice tomatoes, onion and carrot into the oil, and push garlic through a press into the mixture. Add red pepper and vinegar, and sauté for 5 minutes. Add parsley and continue cooking over low heat for 10 minutes. Stir occasionally to prevent sticking. Push the sauce through a fine strainer, pressing all the pulp through and separating only seeds and skins. Add salt and pepper if needed. MAKES ABOUT 2 CUPS.

EGGPLANT AND MEAT SAUCE
For Pasta

TIME: 15 MINUTES
SERVINGS: 6 (½ CUP)
CALORIES: 130 PER ½ CUP

    2 eggplants, 12 ounces each
    6 to 8 shallots
    2 tablespoons olive oil
    2 garlic cloves, peeled
    ¼ cup chopped fresh Italian parsley
    ⅓ teaspoon Italian seasoning
    ⅓ teaspoon crushed red pepper
    ½ pound lean beef, ground
       salt and pepper

Wash and peel eggplants and cut into small dice. Peel and chop shallots; there should be ⅓ cup. Heat oil in a large skillet and push garlic through a press into the oil. Add shallots, eggplant dice, parsley, Italian seasoning and red pepper. Sauté, turning often, until shallots are translucent and eggplant cooked. Add beef and mix and mash it into the vegetables. Sauté until beef loses its red color and is cooked to your taste. Season with salt and pepper to taste. Serve with thicker types of pasta—noodles or larger tubular pasta. MAKES ABOUT 3 CUPS.

VARIATIONS: Add ¼ cup dry red wine, or 1 cup chopped fresh plum tomatoes, for the last minutes of cooking the sauce.

CHICKEN-LIVER SAUCE, IL BOSCHETTO, BRONX, NEW YORK
For Pasta or Plain Rice

      TIME: 15 MINUTES
  SERVINGS: 10 (ABOUT ½ CUP EACH)
  CALORIES: 180 PER ½ CUP

    2 pounds fresh chicken livers
    6 fresh mushrooms
    4 plum tomatoes
    6 to 8 shallots
    1 tablespoon vegetable oil
    1 teaspoon crumbled dried sage
    ⅓ cup chopped fresh Italian parsley
    ½ cup dry white wine

Rinse chicken livers, trim if necessary, and cut into small pieces the size of lima beans. Wash and trim mushrooms and chop; there should be ½ cup.

Wash tomatoes, discard hard portion near stem, and dice; there should be ½ cup. Peel and mince shallots; there should be ⅓ cup. Heat the oil in a large skillet and sauté shallots and mushrooms in it until shallots are translucent and mushrooms browned. Add livers, sage and half of the parsley and sauté, turning often, until livers are no longer pink. Add wine, simmer for a few minutes, then add tomatoes and remaining parsley. Cook for 4 minutes. This sauce is thick; if you prefer it thinner, add more tomatoes and/or wine. MAKES ABOUT 5 CUPS SAUCE.

WHITE-WINE AND DILL SAUCE
For Cooking Fish

TIME: 5 MINUTES
SERVINGS: 4 (¼ CUP EACH)
CALORIES: 27 PER ¼ CUP

> ½ cup dry white wine
> 3 shallots, minced
> ¼ cup chopped fresh dill
> 3 sprigs of Italian parsley, snipped
>   salt and pepper

Mix wine, shallots and herbs in a small bowl. Add salt and pepper to taste. Spoon over raw fish or shellfish before cooking. MAKES ABOUT 1 CUP.

VARIATIONS: Add to the sauce 3 tablespoons prepared mustard; ¼ cup lemon juice; ¼ cup chopped fresh mushrooms or fresh fennel or diced pimientos; or 1 tablespoon capers.

WHITE CLAM SAUCE
For Pasta or Risotto

TIME: 18 MINUTES, EXCLUDING TIME FOR OPENING FRESH CLAMS
SERVINGS: 4 (½ CUP EACH)
CALORIES: 107 PER ½ CUP

1 tablespoon olive oil
1 medium-size onion, chopped
½ garlic clove, peeled
1 cup chopped raw clams with natural juice
½ cup dry white wine
¼ cup chopped fresh Italian parsley
salt and pepper

Heat the oil in a saucepan over low heat, and add chopped onion. Push garlic through a press into the pan, and sauté until onion is translucent, stirring often. Add clams and cook for 3 minutes. Add wine and parsley and simmer for 10 minutes. Season with salt and pepper to your taste. MAKES ABOUT 2 CUPS.

VARIATION: If fresh clams are not available to use, use canned minced clams with their juice. The flavor will be somewhat different, but it will be good. However, since canned clams are already cooked, reduce the cooking time by adding the wine and parsley with the clams and cooking for 8 minutes only.

TO OPEN CLAMS

If you have raw clams in the shell, hold the clam with the hinged part in the hand and insert a clam knife; move the knife around close to the shell until the muscle is cut. If this is new to you, it's easier if the clams have been in the freezer for an hour. Also, for a novice a glove is a help if you're opening more than a dozen. If none of these suggestions gives you any joy, steam the clams to open them, but only for a few minutes so they are not overcooked. However you open the clams, save any juices and let them drip through a strainer to eliminate any tiny bits of shell.

SEAFOOD SAUCE

TIME: 6 TO 10 MINUTES
SERVINGS: 4 (6 TABLESPOONS EACH)
CALORIES: 105 PER 6 TABLESPOONS

   1 *tablespoon vegetable oil*
   3 *shallots, peeled*
   1 *garlic clove, peeled*
   3 *sprigs of Italian parsley*
   1 *teaspoon crushed hot red pepper (optional)*
   2 *teaspoons Italian seasoning*
   1 *cup chopped fresh shrimps, or peeled calamari rings, or*
      steamed fresh tuna, or shelled steamed mussels, or chopped
      fresh scallops
   ½ *cup dry white wine*

Pour oil into a large saucepan. Chop shallots and garlic into the pan. Snip in the parsley and add hot pepper (if you wish) and Italian seasoning. Sauté over medium heat for a few minutes, then add the seafood and wine and cook for 3 minutes. Serve at once. Don't reheat this sauce, as reheating will toughen shrimps, calamari, mussels and scallops. MAKES ABOUT 1½ CUPS.

VARIATION: For red sauce, add ½ cup chopped peeled fresh tomatoes when adding the seafood and wine.

GUIDO'S TUNA AND TOMATO SAUCE
For Pasta and Risotto

TIME: 15 MINUTES
SERVINGS: 10 (¼ CUP EACH)
CALORIES: 63 PER ¼ CUP

   7 *ounces canned water-packed tuna*
   3 *tablespoons grated lemon rind*
   ½ *pound fresh plum tomatoes*
   2 *tablespoons olive oil*
   6 *large shallots, peeled*
   ¼ *cup chopped fresh Italian parsley*
      salt and pepper

Drain tuna and mash in a bowl. Sprinkle lemon rind over the tuna; this counteracts any "fishy" taste. Wash tomatoes and remove hard portion near stem. Chop tomatoes; there should be about 1 cup. Heat oil in a skillet and chop shallots into the pan. Sauté until shallots are translucent. Add tomatoes and parsley, and cook for 5 minutes, stirring. Add tuna and lemon rind and cook for 2 minutes. Season with salt and pepper to taste. MAKES ABOUT 2½ CUPS.

    This is good with green or white fettuccine and ziti. The sauce can be cooked with rice instead of being served over it.

MARSALA SAUCE I
For Chicken, Beef, Veal

TIME:	5 MINUTES
SERVINGS:	4 (2½ TABLESPOONS EACH)
CALORIES:	67 PER 2½ TABLESPOONS

  ½ cup sweet Marsala wine
     juice of ½ lemon
  ½ tablespoon unsalted butter
  1 teaspoon cornstarch

Pour 2 tablespoons of the wine into a small cup and the rest into a small saucepan. Add lemon juice and butter to the saucepan and place over low heat. Stir cornstarch into the 2 tablespoons wine and stir to dissolve starch. When sauce mixture is warm, stir in cornstarch, stirring all the time, until sauce is smooth and thickened. MAKES ABOUT 10 TABLESPOONS.

    Wine, lemon and butter can be used without thickening for a thin sauce.

MARSALA SAUCE II
For Desserts

TIME:	5 MINUTES
SERVINGS:	4 (2½ TABLESPOONS EACH)
CALORIES:	62 PER 2½ TABLESPOONS

  ½ cup sweet Marsala wine
     juice of ½ lemon
  1 tablespoon brandy or Grand Marnier liqueur

Heat ingredients just enough to blend well. Use as a cooking sauce, or serve over completed desserts. MAKES ABOUT 10 TABLESPOONS.

CAPER DRESSING
For Salad, Fish, Veal, Cold Vegetables

TIME: 5 MINUTES
SERVINGS: 8 (3 TABLESPOONS EACH)
CALORIES: 65 PER 3 TABLESPOONS

 2 hard-cooked eggs, shelled
 ½ cup red-wine vinegar
 ¼ teaspoon white pepper
 3 tablespoons vegetable oil
 2 tablespoons chopped capers
 1 garlic clove, peeled and crushed
    dash of Tabasco
    salt and pepper

Mash the eggs and put in a blender container with all other ingredients except salt and pepper. Blend for 2 seconds, until well mixed and smooth. Add salt and pepper to taste. Chill. MAKES ABOUT 1½ CUPS.

PARMESAN DRESSING
For Vegetables

TIME: 10 MINUTES
SERVINGS: 4 (¼ CUP EACH)
CALORIES: 130 PER ¼ CUP

 ¼ cup vinegar
 ¼ cup grated Parmesan cheese
 ¼ cup minced pimiento
 3 tablespoons vegetable oil
 1 garlic clove, put through a press
    salt and pepper

Mix first 5 ingredients in a bowl or bottle, and add salt and pepper to taste. Chill to serve cold, or heat in a small saucepan to serve hot. MAKES ABOUT 1 CUP.

This is excellent cold served over chicory. Wash and trim the chicory and shred or cut into small pieces.

For a hot dish, use artichoke hearts, asparagus, green beans, broccoli, Brussels sprouts, fennel, tomatoes or zucchini. Wash and trim whatever vegetable you are using, and cut into small pieces. Steam until just tender, then serve with the hot Parmesan dressing.

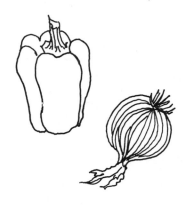

PEPPER AND ONION DRESSING

TIME: 6 MINUTES
SERVINGS: 8 (3 TABLESPOONS EACH)
CALORIES: 45 PER 3 TABLESPOONS

½ cup vinegar
3 tablespoons vegetable oil
¼ teaspoon paprika
3 tablespoons chopped shallots
1 garlic clove, crushed
3 tablespoons chopped green pepper
2 tablespoons chopped fresh Italian parsley
2 tablespoons chopped fresh dill
3 tablespoons prepared Dijon mustard
½ teaspoon Tabasco
   salt

Mix all the ingredients, with salt to taste, in a bowl or bottle. Chill. Serve over a variety of mixed greens or vegetables. MAKES ABOUT 1½ CUPS.

TONNATO DRESSING
For Veal, Fish, Pasta

TIME: 10 MINUTES
SERVINGS: 10 (3 TABLESPOONS EACH)
CALORIES: 60 PER 3 TABLESPOONS

 7 ounces canned water-packed tuna
 2 tablespoons vegetable oil
   juice of 2 lemons
 3 tablespoons chopped fresh Italian parsley
 2 tablespoons capers
 2 shallots, peeled and chopped
 1 tablespoon prepared Dijon mustard

Drain tuna, and flake in a bowl; set aside. Put remaining ingredients in a blender container, and add flaked tuna. Blend for a few seconds, until smooth. Chill. MAKES ABOUT 2 CUPS.

LEMON DRESSING
For Salads, Fish, Cold Veal

TIME: 5 MINUTES
SERVINGS: 6 (4 TEASPOONS EACH)
CALORIES: 48 PER 4 TEASPOONS

 6 tablespoons fresh lemon juice (about 2 lemons)
 2 tablespoons olive oil
   salt and pepper

Pour lemon juice and oil into a cup or small bowl and mix with a whisk until emulsified. Pour dressing over salad, and toss well. Add salt and freshly ground black pepper to taste. Proportions of lemon juice to oil can be changed to taste, but the calorie count will change accordingly. MAKES ½ CUP.

VARIATION: Add minced fresh herbs—basil, parsley or your choice—to dressing just before spooning it over salad.

VINAIGRETTE DRESSING

TIME: 5 MINUTES
SERVINGS: 4 (1½ TABLESPOONS EACH)
CALORIES: 23 PER TABLESPOON

1 *tablespoon vegetable oil*
2 *tablespoons red-wine vinegar*
½ *tablespoon prepared Dijon mustard*
1 *tablespoon snipped fresh dill*
¼ *teaspoon Italian seasoning*
2 *shallots, peeled and minced*
   salt and pepper

The ingredients can be mixed all together, but a better way to dress a salad is to pour the oil into the greens first and toss well. Then mix remaining ingredients, and pour over salad, and toss again. MAKES ABOUT 6 TABLE-SPOONS.

SALSA ALLA TERESA
Vinegar Sauce for Fish, Chicken, Veal

TIME: 15 MINUTES
SERVINGS: 4 (1½ TABLESPOONS EACH)
CALORIES: 42 PER TABLESPOON

3 *tablespoons vinegar*
2 *tablespoons vegetable oil*
1 *garlic clove, peeled*
2 *tablespoons chopped fresh Italian parsley*
½ *teaspoon crumbled dried orégano*
   salt and pepper

Put vinegar and oil in a bowl, and push garlic through a press into the mixture. Add parsley, orégano, and salt and pepper to taste. Beat with a fork for 3 minutes, until well emulsified. Serve at room temperature or cold. MAKES ABOUT 6 TABLESPOONS.

DESSERTS

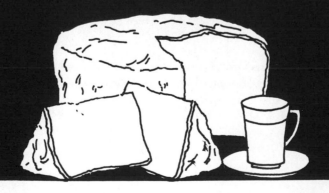

Fruit and cheese is the most popular finish to a meal for the Italians, but they do love special sweets for special occasions, and *gelato*, ice cream. Ice cream in Italy is different from the American product; the milk is different and so are the fruits, picked at their point of perfect ripeness. *Gelato* is sweeter but lighter, with less fat, and one can sample one or two a day without gaining weight.

There are also special *tortas* (layered cakes), pastries and creams. Many classic desserts made for special occasions are elaborate and rich; it would be impossible to adapt them for low-calorie cooking because the fattening ingredients are important to the taste or character of the dish. If you are offered these splendid *dolci* in a home or restaurant, just taste or eat only a small amount.

This chapter presents a variety of fruit desserts as well as some classic preparations that are lighter in calories than the originals that inspired them. Even though these fancies make a perfect ending for a meal, so do fruits, and they are a good choice for everyday occasions.

BAKED FRUIT

Fruits to be baked whole should not be peeled; without the skin they lose their shape during baking. Wash the fruit and remove the stem end. Remove the seed portion from apples with an apple corer, or cut out the stones of peaches or nectarines. Fill the empty space with other fruits, chopped or puréed, or ricotta flavored with Marsala or cinnamon. Place fruits in a shallow baking pan and pour over them a mixture of lemon juice and water or Marsala Sauce II; do not cover the pan. Set in a preheated 350°F. oven, and bake for 10 minutes, or until tender enough for your taste; the kind of fruit and the ripeness of the fruit will determine the cooking time. Apples will take longer than peaches, for instance. Baste often during the baking with the liquid in the bottom of the pan. Allow 1 fruit per serving.

PROPORTIONS

   4 *apples, pears, peaches, or nectarines*
   6 *tablespoons chopped or puréed fruit, or*
   6 *tablespoons skim-milk ricotta cheese mixed with 2 tablespoons*
       Marsala wine or 1 teaspoon ground cinnamon
   1 *cup water mixed with ¼ cup lemon juice, or 1 ¼ cups Marsala*
       Sauce II (p. 250)

FRUIT PURÉES

TIME: 10 MINUTES
SERVINGS: 4
CALORIES: 60 TO 80 DEPENDING ON THE FRUIT USED

Portions of fruit purée can be served as a side dish in the place of a vegetable. With fruits use no eggs or onions, and no herbs or spices.

According to the fresh fruit you may need to peel or to remove pits or seeds or cores. Chop the fruit and put in the blender container. Add ricotta or cottage cheese. Blend to a purée. Good fruits to use are apples, apricots, bananas, cherries, oranges, pineapple, raspberries, strawberries.

These purées make excellent sauces for main courses and desserts. Use your imagination to combine two or more fruits for unusual different tastes.

When preparing these for desserts or dessert sauces, add 2 to 3 tablespoons Marsala wine or Grand Marnier when adding the cheese.

PROPORTIONS
1 cup diced fresh fruit or whole ripe berries
½ cup skim-milk ricotta or cottage cheese
2 tablespoons sweet Marsala wine or Grand Marnier liqueur

ICED FRUIT CREMA

Make a fruit purée following preceding recipe, and freeze it for a dessert similar to a low-calorie ice cream.

FRUIT MOUSSE

TIME: 15 MINUTES, EXCLUDING TIME FOR CHILLING
SERVINGS: 4
CALORIES: 80 PER SERVING

1 cup chopped or puréed fresh fruit without peels or seeds
½ cup skim-milk ricotta cheese
3 tablespoons Grand Marnier liqueur
3 egg whites
½ teaspoon cream of tartar

Put fruit and ricotta in a saucepan and cook over low heat, stirring often, until very smooth. Remove from heat and stir in the Grand Marnier. Let the fruit cool completely. (Set the saucepan in a larger pan filled with ice cubes if you are in a hurry.) Beat egg whites with cream of tartar until stiff. Gently fold into the cooled fruit mixture until well mixed; some tiny flakes of white may show. Spoon the mousse into a 4-cup serving bowl or soufflé dish and chill until set. Serve from the bowl or dish; it will not be firm enough to unmold and still hold its shape.

BAKED STRAWBERRY MOUSSE

TIME: 35 MINUTES
SERVINGS: 4
CALORIES: 80 PER SERVING

Make Fruit Mousse (preceding recipe) using only strawberries. Carefully spoon into a 4-cup soufflé dish and bake in a preheated 350°F. oven for 20 minutes.

FRUIT IN GRAND MARNIER CREME

This dessert can be made ready ahead of time, or can be prepared after the salad has been served and while the espresso pot is boiling. It looks rich, but it is light and delicious.

TIME: 10 MINUTES
SERVINGS: 4
CALORIES: 110 PER SERVING

>   *fruit: 1 apple, ripe pear, peach, orange or banana, or ½ pound*
>   *strawberries or raspberries or pineapple*
> 7 *tablespoons Grand Marnier liqueur*
> ½ *cup skim-milk ricotta cheese*
> ¼ *cup prepared black coffee*
>   *juice of ½ lemon*
> 2 *tablespoons diced strawberries*

Wash the fruit; it can be peeled or prepared with skin. Use one kind or a mixture of fruits. Cut the fruit into very thin slices or small pieces. Pour 4 tablespoons of the Grand Marnier into a cold frying pan of medium size. Turn the ricotta cheese into a small saucepan and add it to the remaining 3 tablespoons Grand Marnier and the black coffee. Set the saucepan over very low heat. Add the prepared fruit to the Grand Marnier in the frying pan and set that pan also over low heat. Gently stir the fruit and liqueur and at the same time constantly stir the cheese mixture over low heat until it becomes a smooth and velvety creme, about 3 minutes. Increase heat under the fruit to medium and cook rapidly for about 4 minutes. Spoon the hot fruit into individual dessert dishes, or into a large bowl. Sprinkle with the lemon juice, then spoon the sauce over the fruit. Top each dish with some of the diced strawberries.

VARIATIONS: When the fruit has been warmed in the liqueur, ignite it and gently stir until flames die down. Serve at once, with the sauce separate.

Instead of Grand Marnier, use kirsch. Serve this without the sauce.

Instead of diced strawberries, spoon raspberry purée on top for a finish.

Instead of ricotta sauce, use a fruit purée mixed with liqueur. (However, if the fruit purée is sweetened, it may not be as low in calories as the ricotta sauce.)

Make the sauce in advance and freeze it. Serve the hot fruit with the cold sauce.

The fruit and the kind of liqueur you choose will vary the taste of the dessert.

The ricotta mixture can be prepared cold, without heating. Use a whisk or rotary beater to make it as smooth as possible, and serve cold.

BERRIES IN SPICED WINE SAUCE

TIME: 10 MINUTES, EXCLUDING TIME FOR CHILLING
SERVINGS: 8
CALORIES: 75 PER SERVING

  ¾ tablespoon ground cinnamon
  1 whole clove
  2 tablespoons lemon juice
  ¾ cup dry red wine
  1 quart fresh strawberries
  1 quart fresh raspberries
  ½ teaspoon sugar or honey (optional)

Put spices, lemon juice and wine in a saucepan and heat for a few minutes; cool. Wash and hull strawberries; drain well. Unless strawberries are very tiny, dice them. Wash raspberries; drain well. Add berries to spiced wine and gently mix. Add sugar or honey if you use it. Cool, chill and serve, plain or as a dessert sauce.

PEACHES IN BAROLO WINE

TIME: 5 MINUTES, EXCLUDING TIME FOR CHILLING
SERVINGS: 6
CALORIES: 55 PER SERVING

        6 *large fresh peaches*
           juice of ½ lemon
        ½ *tablespoon sugar*
        4 *ounces Barolo wine*

Wash peaches, cut into halves, and remove pits. Do not peel peaches, but slice them into a large bowl. Add lemon juice, sugar and wine. Chill. For best results, prepare this before you start the rest of the meal, because it's best when well chilled.

VARIATIONS: Serve in large wine goblets for best appearance.
        Serve over plain cake or ice cream.

PEARS LEONE

TIME: 15 MINUTES, EXCLUDING TIME FOR CHILLING
SERVINGS: 8
CALORIES: 90 PER SERVING

        1 *envelope (7 grams) unflavored gelatin*
        ½ *cup water*
        4 *large ripe pears*
           juice of 2 lemons
        ¼ *cup kirsch liqueur*
        4 *egg whites*
        1 *tablespoon sugar*

Soften gelatin in the ½ cup water. Peel the pears, cut into pieces, and sprinkle the pieces with lemon juice. Put pear pieces and lemon juice in a blender container and purée for a few seconds. Add softened gelatin and purée with the pears. Add kirsch to the purée and mix well. Beat the egg whites with the sugar in a large bowl until stiff. Gently fold the pear and gelatin purée into the egg whites. Chill and serve.

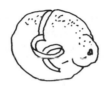

PINEAPPLE CREAM MARNIER

TIME: 10 MINUTES, EXCLUDING TIME FOR CHILLING
SERVINGS: 4
CALORIES: 80 PER SERVING

   1 ½ pounds fresh pineapple
     3 tablespoons Grand Marnier liqueur
       juice of ½ lemon
   ½ cup skim-milk ricotta cheese

Peel and trim the pineapple and cut into small dice. Mix everything in a large bowl until smooth. Chill.

    Blender method: For a very smooth sauce texture, process in a blender; use as a sauce, spooned over cake or a fruit dessert. Or chill in individual serving dishes and serve as a dessert on its own.

VARIATIONS: Canned unsweetened crushed pineapple can be used if fresh pineapple is not available.

    Diced strawberries, or strawberry or raspberry purée, can be added for color.

    Yogurt can be substituted for ricotta.

    The amount of fresh pineapple needed for this recipe, about 2 cups after dicing, is about half of the average market pineapple. You can use the entire pineapple to make a double recipe and store the balance of the recipe in refrigerator or freezer for another occasion.

PINEAPPLE WITH KIRSCH

TIME: 10 MINUTES, EXCLUDING TIME FOR MACERATING
SERVINGS: 8
CALORIES: 80 PER SERVING

1 fresh pineapple, 3 pounds
½ cup kirsch liqueur
juice of 1 lemon

Cut up the pineapple, discard peel and core, and cut the fruit into chunks; there should be at least 4 cups of pieces. Heat kirsch with lemon juice to blend flavors; cool. Pour over pineapple chunks in a glass or pottery bowl and let the fruit macerate for 30 minutes or longer; turn over several times to distribute liqueur. Serve plain, or spooned over plain cake or ice cream.

RASPBERRY SUPREMA

TIME: 10 MINUTES
SERVINGS: 6
CALORIES: 195 PER SERVING

1 pint vanilla ice cream
1 pint fresh raspberries
¼ cup Cointreau
juice of 1 lemon
1 tablespoon sugar

Divide the ice cream among 6 deep dessert plates. Use half of the raspberries to cover the ice cream. Turn remaining raspberries into a small saucepan and add Cointreau, lemon juice and sugar. Heat until sugar is dissolved and sauce well mixed, then pour over ice cream and serve at once.

VARIATION: Use the raspberry sauce over peaches, apricots or strawberries.

STRAWBERRY-FILLED ORANGES

TIME: 15 MINUTES
SERVINGS: 8 (1 ORANGE HALF EACH)
CALORIES: 40 PER HALF-ORANGE

    4 navel oranges
    2 egg whites
    1 quart strawberries
    3 tablespoons Grand Marnier liqueur
    3 tablespoons orange juice
    1 tablespoon grated orange rind
        juice of 1 lemon
    ½ teaspoon ground ginger

Cut oranges into halves and remove pulp. Use the pulp for something else. Beat the egg whites lightly. Brush the inside of each orange shell with egg white. Wash and hull the strawberries and spoon them into the orange shells. Mix remaining ingredients in a bowl, and divide evenly among the strawberry-filled orange halves. Chill.

FRUIT FLAMBÉ ENNIO

TIME: 15 MINUTES
SERVINGS: 6
CALORIES: 195 PER SERVING

    1 small apple
    3 fresh peaches or soft pears
    1 banana
    1 small orange
    1 tablespoon unsalted butter
        juice of 1 lemon
    ¼ cup sweet Marsala wine
    1 pint vanilla ice cream
    ¼ cup Cognac

Wash apple and peaches or pears, cut out stem and blossom ends, and cut into halves. Cut out cores, and cut fruits into thin slices. Peel banana and orange and cut these fruits also into thin slices. Heat the butter in a large frying pan or flambé pan, and add sliced fruits and lemon juice. Toss fruits in the hot butter for a few minutes. Add wine and stir over medium heat for 3 minutes. Divide ice cream among 6 deep dessert dishes. Heat Cognac, pour into fruits, and ignite. When flame dies out, spoon fruit mixture over ice cream and serve immediately.

VARIATION: Use fresh apricots, cherries, pineapple or strawberries instead of any of the fruits listed in the basic recipe.

CAFFÈ MERINGO

TIME: 25 TO 30 MINUTES
SERVINGS: 4 (2 MERINGUES EACH)
CALORIES: 20 PER INDIVIDUAL MERINGUE

    4 *egg whites*
    ½ *teaspoon cream of tartar*
    ¼ *cup instant coffee powder*
    2 *tablespoons coffee liqueur (Tia Maria, Kahlúa)*

Beat egg whites with cream of tartar until stiff peaks remain when the beater is withdrawn. Gently fold in the instant coffee powder and the coffee liqueur. Line a cookie sheet with wax paper. Spoon heaping tablespoons of the meringue onto the wax paper, and make a small depression in the center of each mound. Bake in a preheated 300°F. oven for 15 to 20 minutes, until the meringues are crisp but still pale. MAKES ABOUT 8 MERINGUES.
    Serve with a fruit purée sauce, or a fruit ice or ice cream.

UNBAKED CAFFÈ MERINGO WITH FRUIT

TIME: 10 MINUTES, EXCLUDING TIME FOR CHILLING
SERVINGS: 4
CALORIES: 50 PER SERVING

    4 *egg whites*
    ½ *teaspoon cream of tartar*
    5 *tablespoons instant coffee powder*
    2 *tablespoons coffee liqueur (Tia Maria, Kahlúa)*
    ½ *cup fresh raspberries or diced hulled strawberries*

Beat egg whites with cream of tartar until stiff peaks remain when the beater is withdrawn. Gently fold in the instant coffee powder and the coffee liqueur. Add the fruit to the unbaked meringue, and chill.

COLD APRICOT SOUFFLÉ

TIME: 10 MINUTES, EXCLUDING TIME FOR CHILLING
SERVINGS: 8
CALORIES: 60 PER SERVING

1 *envelope (7 grams) unflavored gelatin*
1 *cup liquid skim milk*
2 *eggs, separated*
1 *cup puréed cooked fresh apricots*
2 *tablespoons Grand Marnier liqueur*
1 *teaspoon almond extract*

Soften gelatin in milk in a large saucepan. Beat egg yolks until lemon-colored and add to milk. Place over low heat or hot water and cook, stirring, until gelatin is dissolved and mixture thickens. Remove from heat and cool.

Add puréed apricots, Grand Marnier and almond extract. As the mixture begins to set, beat the egg whites until stiff. Carefully fold egg whites into the apricot mixture. Spoon into a 4-cup bowl or soufflé dish, or a mold, and chill until firm. Serve plain, or with additional apricot purée mixed with Grand Marnier.

COLD LEMON SOUFFLÉ

TIME: 10 MINUTES, EXCLUDING TIME FOR CHILLING
SERVINGS: 8
CALORIES: 45 PER SERVING

2 *teaspoons unflavored gelatin*
1 ¼ *cups liquid skim milk*
2 *eggs, separated*
¼ *cup fresh lemon juice*
2 *teaspoons Grand Marnier liqueur*
2 *teaspoons grated lemon rind*

Soften gelatin in milk in a large saucepan. Beat egg yolks until lemon-colored; add lemon juice and Grand Marnier, and stir into milk. Place over low heat or hot water and cook, stirring, until gelatin is dissolved and mixture thickens. Remove from heat and cool. Add lemon rind. Beat egg whites until stiff. Carefully fold egg whites into cooled lemon mixture. Spoon into a 4-cup bowl or soufflé dish, and chill until firm. Accompany with fruit if you like.

RICOTTA BRANDY CAFFÈ

TIME: 5 MINUTES, EXCLUDING TIME FOR CHILLING
SERVINGS: 4
CALORIES: 60 PER SERVING

  ½ cup skim-milk ricotta cheese
  5 tablespoons prepared black espresso coffee, cold
  1 tablespoon finely ground dark-roast espresso coffee
  2 tablespoons brandy
  2 tablespoons Grand Marnier liqueur

Put everything in a bowl and whip until smooth. Or process in a blender. Chill. Serve in small dessert dishes, accompanied with cookies and freshly brewed espresso coffee.

VARIATIONS: Add small bits of fruit to the mixture. Serve as a sauce with other desserts.

STRAWBERRY FLUFF AMARETTO

TIME: 15 MINUTES, EXCLUDING TIME FOR CHILLING
SERVINGS: 6
CALORIES: 35 PER SERVING

  3 egg whites, at room temperature
  ¼ teaspoon cream of tartar
  ¼ teaspoon vanilla extract
  2 teaspoons lemon juice
  1 tablespoon Amaretto liqueur
  2 cups diced hulled strawberries

Beat egg whites and cream of tartar with a rotary egg beater, or with an electric mixer at high speed, until stiff. Add vanilla, lemon juice and Amaretto, and continue beating until stiff. At low speed beat in the diced strawberries. Chill.

VARIATION: Top with more strawberries or fresh raspberries or blueberries, or arrange the berries in a ring around the serving of fluff and top with a fresh mint leaf.

FLOATING ISLAND IN AMARETTO SAUCE

TIME: 15 MINUTES
SERVINGS: 4
CALORIES: 110 PER SERVING

¼ cup lemon juice
3 tablespoons water
2 envelopes (7 grams each) unflavored gelatin
4 egg whites
1 teaspoon sugar
½ cup mixed finely sliced fresh fruit (apricots, oranges, peaches, strawberries)
¼ cup Amaretto liqueur

Pour lemon juice and water into a small saucepan. Sprinkle gelatin on top to soften, then heat and stir until gelatin is dissolved. Cool. Beat egg whites with sugar until stiff peaks form when the beater is withdrawn, to make a meringue. Mix fruit with liqueur. Mix dissolved gelatin with fruit, then gently fold the mixture into the meringue. (The lighter meringue floats to the top, making islands in the fruit sauce.) Spoon into individual glasses and chill. Or pour into a 4-cup baking dish and place under the broiler for a few minutes to brown the top, and serve hot. Or serve as a sauce, to spoon over plain cake or ice cream.

DIANA'S COLD ZABAGLIONE

TIME: 20 MINUTES
SERVINGS: 4
CALORIES: 215 PER SERVING

6 *egg yolks*
2 *teaspoons sugar*
½ *cup sweet Marsala wine*
1 *teaspoon espresso coffee powder*
¼ *cup Grand Marnier liqueur*
3 *tablespoons brandy*

Beat egg yolks with sugar for a few minutes. Slowly add the Marsala and beat, then add the coffee powder and mix. Slowly add the Grand Marnier and brandy, and continue to beat until smooth and thick. Chill for 10 minutes. Serve in small wineglasses, or use as a dessert sauce.

FROZEN ZABAGLIONE ALLA MARCO

TIME: 10 MINUTES, EXCLUDING TIME FOR FREEZING
SERVINGS: 4
CALORIES: 90 PER SERVING

3 *eggs*
¼ *cup sweet Marsala wine*
¼ *cup prepared espresso coffee*
2 *teaspoons sugar*

Separate the eggs. Beat yolks lightly, then add Marsala and coffee and beat until well combined. Beat egg whites with the sugar until the meringue forms stiff peaks when beaters are withdrawn. Gently fold meringue into egg-yolk mixture. Divide the mixture among 4 custard cups or other small dessert dishes. Freeze until firm.

FRUIT ICE ALLA GIUSEPPE

TIME: 20 MINUTES
SERVINGS: 4
CALORIES: 80 PER SERVING

1 *cup puréed fresh fruit (peaches, raspberries, strawberries)*
¼ *cup fresh lemon juice*
3 *tablespoons brandy*

Put fruit purée, lemon juice and brandy in a large metal bowl. Set the bowl in a larger container filled with crushed ice. Stir the mixture with a large wire whisk until it is smooth and creamy. (It is never actually frozen.) Serve immediately.

GRAPEFRUIT AND BANANA ICE ALLA TAORMINA

TIME: 20 MINUTES
SERVINGS: 4
CALORIES: 90 PER SERVING

1 *cup puréed fresh grapefruit and banana, mixed half and half*
¼ *cup fresh lemon juice*
3 *tablespoons brandy*

Put fruit purée, lemon juice and brandy in a large metal bowl. Set the bowl in a larger container filled with crushed ice. Stir the mixture with a large wire whisk until it is smooth and creamy. (It is never actually frozen.) Serve immediately.

DESSERT FRITTATA

A full description of Frittata is given on page 185.

TIME: 15 MINUTES, EXCLUDING TIME FOR MACERATING FRUIT
SERVINGS: 6
CALORIES: 150 PER SERVING

6 *eggs*
1 *teaspoon sugar*
3 *tablespoons liqueur*
2 *tablespoons unsalted butter*
½ *cup filling*
3 *tablespoons sweet Marsala*

LIQUEUR: Use Grand Marnier for orange flavor, Amaretto for almond flavor, or brandy.

FILLING: Use apricots, cherries, oranges, peaches, strawberries. Wash or peel or pit, according to the fruit, and cut into thin slices or chop. Pour the Marsala over the prepared fruit and let it macerate for 10 minutes, or longer if you prefer.

Beat eggs lightly with sugar and liqueur; be sure the sugar is dissolved. Heat butter in a large skillet and pour in the egg mixture. Let it cook for a minute, then spoon the fruit mixture into the center and continue to cook over low heat for 4 or 5 minutes, until the top is set.

VARIATIONS: Broil the *frittata* for a minute or two to caramelize the top.

Pour 3 to 4 tablespoons orange or lemon juice over the top.

Instead of spooning the fruit into the center of the eggs, let the sweet *frittata* cook until set, then spoon fruit over the top. Heat 3 to 4 tablespoons brandy or liqueur, pour over the top, ignite it, and serve flaming.

DESSERT FRITTATA WITH MERINGUE

TIME: 20 MINUTES
SERVINGS: 6
CALORIES: 160 PER SERVING

Assemble the ingredients for the Dessert Frittata (preceding recipe) and in addition 3 egg whites. Beat the egg whites with a pinch of salt until stiff peaks remain when the beaters are withdrawn. Heat the butter until foamy, then add the macerated fruit and let it get hot. Spoon the mixture of whole eggs, sugar and liqueur over the fruit and cook until nearly set. Gently spread the meringue over the *frittata*, then finish by baking in a preheated 425°F. oven for 5 minutes, until meringue is golden; or finish under the broiler. This *frittata* can be served hot or cold.

STRAWBERRY FRITTATA

TIME: 20 MINUTES
SERVINGS: 4
CALORIES: 170 PER SERVING

    1 cup fresh strawberries
    2 tablespoons Maraschino liqueur
    4 eggs
    2 tablespoons water
    2 tablespoons unsalted butter
    1 teaspoon confectioners' sugar

Wash and hull strawberries; let them dry, then cut them into halves. Put them in a bowl with a tight-fitting cover and add Maraschino. Cover and refrigerate for 10 minutes. Shake or stir the berries several times so all are flavored and sweetened with the liqueur. Beat eggs and water together. Heat butter in a skillet; when it is foaming, add eggs and cook over low heat for 3 minutes, until *frittata* is lightly browned on the bottom. Cover the pan and cook for 3 minutes longer, until the top is set. Slide *frittata* onto a round serving plate, spoon berries over the top, and sprinkle with confectioners' sugar. Cut into wedges to serve.

SCARPELLAS
Dessert Pancakes

TIME: 20 TO 25 MINUTES, EXCLUDING TIME FOR RESTING BATTER
SERVINGS: 8 (2 PANCAKES EACH)
CALORIES: 70 PER SERVING, EXCLUDING FILLING

    ¼ cup unbleached flour
    ½ teaspoon sugar
    1 cup liquid skim milk
    3 eggs
    1 tablespoon unsalted butter

Mix flour and sugar. Beat milk and eggs together until well mixed but not foamy. Pour into flour and beat with a whisk or wooden spoon until smooth. If possible, let batter rest in a cool place for 30 minutes. Heat a 7-inch crêpe pan or frying pan and melt the butter in it. Pour off the butter into a custard cup and keep it warm; the crêpe pan should have only a thin coating of butter. Spoon 2 tablespoons of the batter into the hot pan and at once turn and tilt the pan so that batter covers the bottom of the pan, making a very thin layer. Cook for 2 minutes, then flip over and slightly brown the other side, for 1 minute. Remove to a warm plate. Pour butter again into the pan, heat it, then pour off, leaving only a thin coating of butter. Make another pancake in the same fashion as the first, and stack on the warm plate. Continue until batter is all cooked.

To serve, spoon 2 tablespoons filling into the center of each pancake, and roll or fold pancakes over the filling. For party occasions, spoon a little brandy or other liqueur over each *scarpello,* ignite it, and serve flaming.

Filling recipes follow.

ORANGE FILLING
For Scarpellas

TIME: 10 MINUTES
SERVINGS: 8
CALORIES: 160 PER SERVING

  2 *navel oranges*
  ¼ *pound unsalted butter*
     juice of 4 lemons
  ½ *cup Grand Marnier liqueur*

Peel oranges, remove all white interior peel, and with a sharp knife dice orange segments; there should be about 2 cups. Melt butter in a saucepan and heat orange dice and lemon juice in the butter; mix well. Spoon 2 tablespoons of the filling into each pancake and roll or fold them. Pour ½ tablespoon Grand Marnier over each one.

FRUIT FILLING
For Scarpellas

TIME: 10 MINUTES
SERVINGS: 8
CALORIES: 35 PER SERVING

    2 cups chopped fresh fruits (strawberries, peaches, etc.)
    2 tablespoons sweet Marsala wine
      juice of 2 lemons
    2 tablespoons sugar

Use 1 pint fresh strawberries, 4 to 6 fresh peaches or apricots or pears. Wash, hull, remove pits or cores, drain well, and chop. Turn into a saucepan and heat with the wine, lemon juice and sugar until sugar is dissolved and the filling hot. Spoon 2 tablespoons filling into each pancake and roll or fold them.

ICE-CREAM FILLING WITH AMARETTO
For Scarpellas

    TIME: 10 MINUTES
SERVINGS: 8
CALORIES: 130 PER SERVING

    1 pint chocolate, coffee or fruit ice cream
    2 tablespoons brandy
    6 tablespoons prepared black coffee
    ¼ cup Amaretto liqueur

Let ice cream soften until you can stir it. Pour in brandy, coffee and Amaretto, and mix until smooth. If ice cream is too liquid after mixing, chill it before using it. Spoon 2 tablespoons into each cold pancake, roll up, and serve at once. If there is any filling left, spoon it over the tops of the pancakes.

ITALIAN RUM CAKE

    TIME: 15 MINUTES
SERVINGS: 8
CALORIES: 190 PER SERVING

1 baked sponge cake or pound cake, 8 inches square, 1 inch thick
½ cup prepared black coffee
¼ cup rum
1 tablespoon brandy
1 pint fresh strawberries
1 teaspoon sugar
  juice of ½ lemon

Cut cake into 8 pieces and put each piece on a dessert plate. Mix coffee with rum and brandy, then spoon over the cake, a little at a time, until it is all absorbed. Wash and hull strawberries and slice; there should be 2 cups. Sprinkle with the sugar and lemon juice and gently mix to distribute sugar. Spoon strawberries over cake.

VARIATIONS: Instead of strawberries use raspberries, or apricots or peaches.
    A lemon-flavored pudding or custard can be spooned over the cake pieces before the fruit is added (this will add calories).

RICOTTA CAKE ALLA SICILIANA

TIME: 45 MINUTES
SERVINGS: 6
CALORIES: 200 PER SERVING WITH WHOLE-MILK RICOTTA, 180 WITH
              SKIM-MILK

3 eggs
¼ cup sugar
1 pound fresh whole-milk or skim-milk ricotta
3 tablespoons all-purpose flour
  pinch of baking soda
3 tablespoons chopped blanched almonds
*¼ cup diced fresh fruit (apricots, oranges, pineapple or
    strawberries)*
¼ cup grated lemon rind
3 tablespoons Italian brandy
  butter and flour for pan

Beat the eggs with the sugar in a large bowl. Add ricotta and continue to beat. Slowly add the flour and baking soda, then all the other ingredients, continuing to beat until the batter is well mixed and light. Butter and flour a 6-cup springform pan, and with a large spoon transfer batter to the prepared pan. Bake in a preheated 350°F. oven for 30 minutes. Let the cake cool, then run a thin flexible knife or spatula around the mold to loosen the cake. Carefully remove the rim of the springform and slide the cake, still on the bottom of the pan, onto a serving plate. Ricotta cake has a delicate texture, so don't try to remove it from the pan bottom. In fact, if it looks too fragile, serve it from the baking pan. Cut into wedges to serve.

TORTA DI RISO
Rice Cake

TIME: 45 TO 50 MINUTES
SERVINGS: 8
CALORIES: 185 PER SERVING

       3 cups milk
       ½ cup uncooked Italian white rice
       2 teaspoons grated lemon rind
       2 teaspoons sugar
       4 eggs, separated
       ¼ cup Italian brandy
       2 teaspoons Amaretto liqueur
       ¼ cup ground almonds
          butter for mold

Bring milk to a simmer, and slowly pour in the rice. Add lemon rind and sugar. Cook slowly until rice has absorbed the milk. Remove from heat and cool. Preheat oven to 400°F. Beat the egg yolks with brandy and Amaretto, and add to the rice with the almonds. Beat egg whites until stiff peaks form when the beater is withdrawn. Gently fold into the rice mixture. Pour into a buttered 6-cup mold. Bake in the preheated oven for 15 minutes. Serve hot or cold.

VARIATIONS: Add chopped fruit; choose from many varieties.
        Flame the top of the *torta* with brandy just before serving.

RICOTTA CHEESE TORTA WITH FRUIT

TIME: 15 MINUTES, EXCLUDING TIME FOR CHILLING
SERVINGS: 12
CALORIES: 80 CALORIES PER SLICE (MORE WITH ORANGES, LESS WITH
STRAWBERRIES)

2 tablespoons lemon juice
1 envelope (7 grams) unflavored gelatin
½ cup liquid skim milk, hot
1 teaspoon grated orange rind
2 eggs, separated
2½ cups skim-milk ricotta cheese
¼ cup Marsala wine or Grand Marnier liqueur
1 cup crushed ice
2 cups fresh raspberries, strawberries or orange sections

Pour lemon juice into a blender container and sprinkle gelatin on top. Add
hot skim milk, orange rind, egg yolks, ricotta and 2 tablespoons wine or
liqueur. Whip at high speed for 2 seconds. Add ice and run at high speed until
mixture is well blended. Beat egg whites until stiff. Fold into gelatin mixture,
carefully and slowly, with a blending motion. Pour mixture into a 6-cup
oblong pan or large round pan and chill until firm.

Purée the raspberries, strawberries or oranges with remaining wine
or liqueur in the blender for 2 minutes, and serve with the cheese pie. Or
serve the pie plain with fresh strawberries on top.

GRAPE AND APRICOT TART

TIME: 15 MINUTES, EXCLUDING TIME TO PREPARE PIE SHELL
SERVINGS: 8
CALORIES: 225 PER SERVING

1 pound white grapes
6 apricots
¼ cup brandy
3 egg yolks, well beaten
2 tablespoons cornstarch
1 tablespoon sugar
2 cups liquid skim milk, scalded
1 tablespoon vanilla extract
1 baked pie shell, 9-inch size

Wash grapes and roll in a towel to dry. Cut them into halves, and remove seeds. Wash and dry apricots, and cut into small pieces. Put both fruits and the brandy into a bowl with a tight cover and let fruit macerate. Turn the bowl over now and then to distribute the brandy evenly.

In a saucepan mix beaten egg yolks, cornstarch and sugar. Place over low heat. Add milk and vanilla. Cook and stir until thick. Pour custard into the baked pie shell. Arrange grape halves in a circle around the edge, and put apricot pieces in the center. Chill and serve.

WHOLE-WHEAT PIE PASTRY

TIME: 10 MINUTES TO MAKE PASTRY, 1 HOUR TO CHILL, 25
MINUTES TO BAKE
CALORIES: 800 PER PIE SHELL, 175 PER INDIVIDUAL TART SHELL

1 ½ cups whole-wheat flour
½ cup unbleached all-purpose flour
pinch of salt
½ cup vegetable oil
½ cup very cold water

Dump both flours into a large bowl and mix well. Add salt (more if you prefer). Mix oil and water with a fork and dump into the flour all at once. Mix liquids into the flour with the fork or with a wooden paddle until all flour is moistened and the ingredients can be picked up in a ball. Dough will be very moist, but don't be tempted to add more flour, as that makes tough pastry. Divide the dough into portions according to what you plan to do with it. Roll out each portion between sheets of wax paper into a sheet as thin as possible. Remove the top sheet of paper and use the bottom sheet to flip the dough over onto the pan you are using. Pat the dough into the pan, without stretching it, and trim all around the edge with kitchen scissors, allowing about 1 inch excess. Fold the extra inch under the edge all around, and crimp with a fork or flute with fingers. Place the filled pan or pans in the refrigerator for 1 hour.

Preheat oven to 375°F. Line the chilled pastry with foil and fill with raw rice, dried beans, or aluminum pie pellets. Bake for about 12 minutes, then gently remove the foil and weight and return to the oven for 10 minutes longer. Let the crust cool slightly, then fill and finish baking with the filling. Makes enough for two 9-inch pie or tart shells, with some extra pastry, or 8 to 10 individual 4½- to 5-inch tarts.

CALORIE CHARTS

CALORIE CHARTS

No calorie table can offer an exact match for the foods in your market basket; rather, it is a table of potential figures. Products vary by brand, and produce certainly varies by size. The charts are designed to help you plan your shopping and menus. The foods listed are those used in the recipes.

If calories are important to you, you will eventually reach a point where you can look at a food item and it automatically says "yes" or "no" to you. It isn't true that the best-tasting and most exciting foods are inevitably the most fattening, but portions are extremely important. Too much of a low-calorie dish can equal a small amount of a high-calorie food.

If you find yourself at a special function or dinner where everything is rich and elaborate, stay with the moment. Enjoy the meal, the wine, the people, and don't think about dieting. But next day cut down your food consumption and balance the calorie intake over the next few days. Follow neither self-indulgence or self-denial. Moderation is the key.

THE GREAT VEGETABLE NIBBLERS
FOR APÉRITIF FOOD, FIRST COURSE, OR ACCOMPANIMENT TO MAIN COURSE

Raw vegetables are low in calories and provide necessary bulk in the diet. They are good to look at by themselves, and can be presented in various attractive ways. Mix colors and types, and make good flavor combinations. Refrigerate vegetables until time to serve them.

VEGETABLE	AMOUNT	CALORIES
asparagus	1 stalk	4 or 5
broccoli	1 flowering head, 1 ounce	10
carrot	1 carrot, 2 ounces	21
cauliflower	1 floweret, 1 ounce	8
celery	1 large rib	6
cucumber	1 small cucumber, pared	29
fennel	1 rib	3
olives, black	1 small olive	5
olives, green	1 large olive	5
parsley	½ cup sprigs	10
pepper, green	1 pepper without stem, ribs and seeds, 3 ounces	15
pepper, red	1 pepper, without stem, ribs and seeds, 3 ounces	20

VEGETABLE	AMOUNT	CALORIES
radishes	1 large radish	2
scallion (green onion)	1 scallion	4
tomatoes	1 cup cherry tomatoes	42
turnip	½ cup peeled raw strips	15
watercress	5 sprigs	1
zucchini	1 raw round, 1 ounce	5

CALORIES OF MOST-USED FOODS

FOOD	AMOUNT	CALORIES
alcoholic beverages		
beer	12 ounces	150 to 170
distilled spirits (bourbon, gin, Scotch, vodka)	1 ounce, 80 to 100 proof	70 to 85
liqueurs		
brandy	1 ounce	80
Grand Marnier	1 ounce	100
Maraschino	1 ounce	94
Tia Maria, Kahlúa	1 ounce	92
wine		
Champagne, dry	4 ounces	100 to 115
Marsala, dry	4 ounces	160
Marsala, sweet	4 ounces	200
vermouth, dry	4 ounces	135
red wine, dry	4 ounces	95 to 100
white wine, dry	4 ounces	85 to 95
anchovy	1 fillet	7
apple	1 unpeeled apple, 5 ounces	80
artichoke	1 fresh artichoke, 8 ounces	35
	3 frozen hearts	22
asparagus	1 pound	66
beans		
green or wax	½ cup cooked fresh beans	16
Italian	½ cup cooked fresh beans	45
beef		
chuck	3½ ounces, lean, braised	265
club steak	3½ ounces, lean, broiled	280
ground beef	3½ ounces, lean, broiled	220
round, bottom	3½ ounces, lean, broiled	240
steak, lean	3½ ounces raw	164

FOOD	AMOUNT	CALORIES
bouillon cube	1 cube	5
bread		
cracked wheat	1 slice	60
Italian	1 slice, 1 inch thick	55
white	1 slice	70
whole wheat	1 slice	55
broccoli	1 pound raw	113
	½ cup cooked fresh	25
butter	1 tablespoon	100
carrot	½ pound raw	80
cauliflower	½ pound raw	60
celery	1 cup diced raw	15
cheese		
cottage or ricotta	skim-milk, ½ cup	80
mozzarella	1 ounce	80
Parmesan or pecorino	1 tablespoon grated	30
chicken		
breast	3½ ounces raw	100
	3½ ounces, without skin, broiled or poached	135
dark meat	3½ ounces, roasted	180
white meat	3½ ounces, roasted	165
clams	3½ ounces fresh meats	82
	3½ ounces canned meats, drained	98
cod	3½ ounces fresh	78
	3½ ounces salted	130
cornstarch	1 tablespoon	30
crab	3½ ounces fresh	93
	3½ ounces canned	101
crackers		
graham	1 medium-size cracker	28
saltine	1 saltine	22
Venus Wheat Wafers	1 wafer	18
cream, light whipping	1 tablespoon	45
cream, sour	1 tablespoon	30
egg	1 whole large egg	80

FOOD	AMOUNT	CALORIES
	1 large egg white	15
	1 large egg yolk	60
eggplant	3½ ounces raw	25
	½ cup simmered pieces	19
endive and escarole	3½ ounces raw	20
flounder	3½ ounces raw	79
flour		
whole-wheat	3½ ounces hard wheat	333
enriched all-purpose	3½ ounces	364
garlic	1 clove, 3 grams	3
gelatin	1 envelope, 7 grams, unflavored	28
gingerroot	½ ounce fresh	7
grapefruit	½ white grapefruit, 7 ounces	50
	1 cup fresh sections	75
grapes	1 cup raw seedless green grapes	95
haddock	3½ ounces raw	80
halibut	3½ ounces raw	100
honey	1 tablespoon	64
lamb		
leg	3½ ounces lean, roasted	195
loin chop	5 ounces, lean, with bone	225
rib chop	5 ounces, lean, with bone	325
shoulder	3½ ounces lean, roasted	220
leek	1 large raw leek	17
lemon	1 tablespoon fresh juice	4
lettuce		
iceberg	½ pound raw	28
loose-leaf	½ pound raw	26
romaine	½ pound raw	26
liver		
beef	3½ ounces raw	125
	3½ ounces broiled	180
calf's	3½ ounces raw	140
	3½ ounces broiled	220

FOOD	AMOUNT	CALORIES
chicken	3½ ounces raw	110
	3½ ounces simmered	165
lobster		
American	3½ ounces raw meat	91
spiny	3½ ounces raw meat	72
milk		
skim	1 cup, 8 ounces	90
whole	1 cup, 8 ounces	160
mushrooms	½ pound raw	60
mussels	3½ ounces raw meats, no shells	66
mustard	1 tablespoon prepared	11
oil		
olive	1 tablespoon	130
vegetable	1 tablespoon	120 to 130
olives		
black (ripe)	1 small olive	5
green	1 large olive	5
onion	½ pound raw	80
	1 onion, 3 ounces	30
	1 tablespoon chopped raw	4
	½ cup chopped raw	32
orange	1 Florida orange, 7 ounces	75
	1 California orange, 6 ounces	60
oysters	3½ ounces fresh raw meat of Eastern oysters	66
parsley	1 tablespoon chopped	2
pasta	2 ounces uncooked	210
macaroni	½ cup cooked *al dente*, with no sauce	95
noodles	½ cup cooked *al dente*, with no sauce	100
spaghetti	½ cup cooked *al dente*, with no sauce	95
peach	1 fresh peach, 4 ounces	35
pear	1 fresh pear, 7 ounces	100

FOOD	AMOUNT	CALORIES
peas, fresh green	½ cup cooked	57
pepper, sweet bell	1 green pepper, 5 ounces	25
	1 red pepper, 5 ounces	35
pignoli (pine nuts)	1 tablespoon	50
pimiento	1 canned	10
pineapple	½ cup diced fresh	36
	3½ ounces canned, packed in	
	natural juices	58
potato	1 potato, 3½ ounces, raw	78
	1 potato, 3½ ounces, peeled	
	and boiled	65
quail	3½ ounces raw, without skin	
	and bones	168
rabbit	3½ ounces raw, without skin	
	and bones	162
radishes	3½ ounces, 1 cup, about 15	
	small radishes	25
raisins	½ cup	230
raspberries	½ cup fresh raw	35
rice		
white, long-grain	3½ ounces raw	369
	½ cup cooked	92
brown	3½ ounces raw	360
	½ cup cooked	100
rugola	½ pound raw	50
salmon	3½ ounces raw	220
	3½ ounces poached	210
	4 ounces canned	160 to 240
sardines	3½ ounces raw	160
	3½ ounces canned in brine	196
	3½ ounces canned in oil,	
	drained	205
scallions	6 scallions without tops	20
scallops	3½ ounces raw	81
	3½ ounces steamed	112
shallots	1 ounce	18

FOOD	AMOUNT	CALORIES
shrimps	3½ ounces fresh	91
	3½ ounces canned	116
snapper	3½ ounces fresh, without skin or bones	90
soft drinks		
club soda	8 ounces	0
cola	8 ounces	95
ginger ale	8 ounces	85
sole	3½ ounces fresh, without skin or bones	79
spinach	3½ ounces raw	26
	½ cup boiled, drained	21
squash		
yellow summer squash	3½ ounces raw	20
	½ cup cooked, drained	16
zucchini	3½ ounces raw	17
	½ cup cooked, drained	13
squid	3½ ounces raw	84
stock		
chicken	1 cup	30
veal	1 cup	35
vegetable	1 cup	10
strawberries	3½ ounces fresh raw, about ⅔ cup	37
striped bass	3½ ounces raw, without skin and bones	105
sugar		
brown	1 tablespoon	50
white	1 tablespoon	45
tomato paste	canned, 1 tablespoon	15
tomato purée	canned, ¼ cup	24
tomatoes		
cherry tomatoes	1 cup	42
plum tomatoes	1 tomato, 8 to 1 pound	13
	canned, ½ cup	25
round tomatoes	1 tomato, 3 to 1 pound	35

FOOD	AMOUNT	CALORIES
trout	3½ ounces raw fresh brook trout	101
tuna	3½ ounces canned in oil	285
	3½ ounces canned in water	170
turkey	3½ ounces raw white meat, without skin and bones	116
	3½ ounces roasted white meat, without skin and bones	175
veal		
loin chop	6 ounces, with bone, raw	210
scallop *(scaloppine)*	1 scallop, 2 ounces	120
shoulder or rump	3½ ounces, with no fat	163
vinegar	1 tablespoon	2
watercress	3½ ounces	17
	5 sprigs	1
Worcestershire sauce	1 tablespoon	15
yogurt	1 cup, part-skim milk, plain	125

These tables are based on information published by the United States Department of Agriculture. For more nutritional information about these foods, or for information about other foods, consult the USDA handbook *Composition of Foods.*

The mysterious figure "3½ ounces" is the closest equivalent to 100 grams, which is the basic unit used in computing calories. A calorie is a man-made unit used for the amount of heat needed to raise 1 gram of water 1 degree Celsius at a pressure of 1 atmosphere.

GLOSSARY

AL DENTE: to the tooth, that is, with texture to chew, not mushy; used of pasta, rice, vegetables.

ANTIPASTO: before the pasta; appetizer, hors-d'oeuvre, or first course.

APERITIVO: apéritif; a drink, often before a meal, that is usually wine or a fortified or aromatized wine.

ARRABBIATA: lit., furious or raging; used for a sauce made spicy with hot peppers, or for a dish that is prepared with hot peppers (chicken, pasta, etc.).

BLANCH: 1. to dip into boiling water briefly, to remove the skin (almonds, tomatoes). 2. to parboil, to end enzyme action and set the color (vegetables, especially green leafy kinds).

BOIL: to cook in water to cover at a temperature of 212°F.

BRACIOLE: thin slices of meat, usually flattened, filled with a small amount of stuffing, rolled up, and fastened with string or skewers; they are sautéed, then the cooking is finished with wine, stock or sauce.

BRAISE: to cook in moist heat, covered, on top of the stove or in the oven; the amount of moisture is minimal, often only the natural juices of the food to be braised.

CACCIATORA: lit., hunter style; a way of preparing chicken, rabbit or quail; the meat is sautéed, then the cooking is finished with a sauce made of wine, onion and usually a small amount of tomatoes.

CANNELLINI: large white shell beans, like kidney beans; in the United States usually found only canned or dried.

CELERY RIB: one piece, the fleshy base ending in leaves, broken from a stalk; a celery stalk is an entire plant.

CHICKEN BREAST: the entire breast portion of the bird; this divides at the breast bone into two half-breasts; each half-breast has two fillets, a larger and a smaller. All poultry breasts are similar in construction.

CHOLESTEROL: a fat-soluble crystalline steroid alcohol, synthesized in the human body; when there is too much, it is deposited in the blood vessels.

CHOP: to reduce any food to bits of random size; usually all the pieces are less than ½ inch; chopped pieces are larger than minced pieces. Cf. CUBE and DICE.

CLARIFY: 1. to remove all solid particles, however small, from stock for aspic or consommé to give a clear transparent liquid. 2. to separate milky particles from butter to give only the clear butterfat, so that butter will not burn when used for cooking.

CONTORNI: vegetables used as accompaniment to meat, poultry or fish.

CROSTINI: pieces of toast, especially toasts with some sort of topping used for antipasto.

CRUSH: to flatten or mash, usually said of raw foods, especially garlic; garlic is crushed with the flat side of a chef's knife.

CRUSTACEANS: marine creatures with segmented exterior skeletons—crab, lobster, shrimp.

CUBE: to cut into cubes—pieces of equal dimensions on all sides; unless the size is specified, a cube is usually more than ½ inch but less than 1 inch in size. Cf. DICE.

DEVEIN: to remove the intestinal tract of a shrimp.

DICE: to cut into cube-shaped pieces of less than ½ inch; cubes are larger. Both CHOP and MINCE indicate pieces of random size, but dice are all of the same size.

DOLCI: sweets, cakes, etc.; desserts generally.

DOPPIO: double strength, as in consommé concentrated to make it more flavorful and nutritious; like French *consommé double.*

DRAIN: to pour off liquid, which is not retained for future use, as draining cooked pasta; the solid food retained in the colander or strainer is used. Cf. STRAIN.

DRESS: to prepare fish and crustaceans for cooking and eating; each style of preparation has a specific name, as drawn, filleted, pan-dressed, whole-dressed.

DRIED: used for a product that is made dry by artificial heat or by the sun's heat to make it possible to store it for later use, as dried beans, dried apricots, dried herbs.

DRY: used for a product that is dry in its natural mature state, as mustard seeds, whole or ground; hence "dry mustard."

DRY (wine): not sweet; however, all such "flavor" terms are relative.

DURUM SEMOLINA: flour or meal made from the grain *Triticum durum;* the flour, high in gluten-producing proteins, is used for the best pasta.

ENZYME: a substance of the nature of a protein produced by living cells, as in fruits, meats, vegetables, which promotes reactions such as combination with water or oxygen.

ESPRESSO: black coffee made by forcing steam through finely ground dark-roast coffee beans.

FENNEL RIB: see CELERY RIB. A stalk or head of fennel is the whole plant.

FILET: the tenderloin of beef, running through the short loin and sirloin; it is boneless and very tender; similar but much smaller tenderloins are found in other meat animals.

FILET MIGNON: a slice, 1 to 1½ inches thick, cut from the beef filet; one of these weighs 6 to 8 ounces. Cf. TOURNEDOS.

FILLET: 1. the boneless flesh cut from one side of a fish; it may retain the skin or not; larger fish may be divided along the center line to make quartercut fillets.
2. one of the parts of the half-breast of chicken; see CHICKEN BREAST.

FIORENTINA: in the style of Florence. When recipes use the English word "Florentine" it almost always means "with spinach."

FLAKE: to separate cooked fish along its natural lines of division, making small thin flattened pieces; when this can be done with the touch of a fork, the fish is cooked.

FLAMBÉ: to spoon or pour an alcoholic liquid, usually brandy or other high-proof liqueur, over a food and to ignite it; this can be done during cooking or at serving time.

FRITTATA: an egg dish similar to an omelet, but usually cooked on both sides and having any filling mixed into the beaten eggs.

FRITTO: lit., fried; also a dish of fried food.

FRITTO MISTO: a mixed fry; a mixture of different ingredients all fried and served together.

GARLIC CLOVE: one bulblet separated from a head of garlic; before peeling one clove may weigh about ¹⁄₁₀ ounce.

GELATO: ice cream; because Italian ice cream is made with less fat, it is more like an American ice or sherbet.

GLUTEN: a stretchy and tough protein found in wheat flour; to keep piecrust from being tough, it is chilled at some stage to allow the gluten to relax.

GRAND MARNIER: an orange-flavored brandy-based liqueur made in France; the 80-proof yellow liqueur, which is sweeter than the red, is used for sweetening in some of these desserts.

GRATE: to reduce to small particles by rubbing against a grater; the bits can be very small, as when nutmeg is grated, but they are always smaller than shreds. Cf. SHRED.

GRIND: to reduce to small bits in a mechanical grinder, powered by hand or electricity; the size of the bits depends on the size of the holes in the grinding plate. One can also grind by hand using a pestle in a mortar.

HERB: a flavoring ingredient based on the leaves of plants of temperate climates; there are a few seed herbs, and garlic (a bulb) and horseradish (a root) are also counted as herbs. Cf. SPICE.

LEGUMI: legumes; peas, beans, etc., used fresh in pods or fresh shelled or dried shelled.

LEMON RIND: the outer yellow portion of the peel; this contains the aromatic lemon oil. It is usually grated for use; in this state it can be dried or frozen for future use.

LIMONE: lemon in Italian.

MACERATE: to soak fruits in an acid (lemon juice or wine) or a liqueur, to soften and flavor them.

MARINATE: to soak meat, poultry, fish, occasionally vegetables, in an acid (wine, vinegar, lemon juice) and various flavorings to tenderize and flavor it.

MERINGO: meringue in Italian.

MINCE: to reduce to very tiny pieces of random size by chopping; esp. said of parsley and other herbs. Cf. CHOP.

MINERAL: one of several chemical elements essential to life, found in foods in varying amounts; some that we know to be necessary to us are iron, calcium, potassium, phosphorus.

MINESTRA: soup, generally thick, made of vegetables and often including a small variety of pasta.

MINESTRINA: a thin clear soup, like consommé.

MINESTRONE: a thick vegetable soup, also containing either rice or pasta.

MISTO: mixture in Italian; as in *fritto misto,* a "mixed fry."

MONOUNSATURATED: able to form only one addition product with another nutrient; olive oil is an example. Cf. POLYUNSATURATED.

MOUSSE: a dish made of puréed food mixed with cream (or cream substitute) and sometimes gelatin; a mousse can be a dessert or a main dish or first course; it can be chilled or frozen, or it can be baked; usually a mousse is too soft-textured to be unmolded, but there are exceptions.

MOZZARELLA: lit., cheese that can be cut; a mild moist cheese, good for eating plain or in cooked dishes; in the U.S.A. made of cow's milk.

OIL-STEAM: to steam with a small amount of oil, the rest of the needed moisture being supplied by the ingredients being cooked; esp. for vegetables.

PARMESAN: lit., of Parma; an aged grainy cheese produced in a strictly delimited area of Italy; it is an excellent eating cheese when young, but is more used as a flavoring cheese when well aged; true Parmigiano-Reggiano is not exported until aged for two years.

PASTA ASCIUTTA: dry pasta, the kind one buys in packages in the market.

PASTA FRESCA: pasta freshly made at home, usually cooked soon after.

PASTA IN BRODO: small pasta shapes, cooked and served in broth.

PASTINA: tiny pasta shapes, especially for *pasta in brodo.*

PAVESE: lit., of Pavia; decorated; used of soup garnished with a whole poached egg on a piece of fried bread or toast.

PECORINO: cheese made of ewe's milk; this is aged for grating just as Parmesan is; Pecorino Romano is the most familiar kind in the U. S. A.

PESTO: lit., pounded or bruised; the name of a sauce made with fresh basil leaves, grated cheese and olive oil, sometimes with additional ingredients. Originally the ingredients were pounded in a mortar with a pestle.

PIAZZIOLA: lit., in the style of the piazza or marketplace; a sauce for cooking meat, made of tomatoes, herbs and sometimes other vegetables.

PICCANTE: lit., piquant; appetizing, spicy, with a slight hot taste from hot peppers, ginger or cayenne.

PIGNOLI: pine nuts, the seeds of several varieties of pine trees.

PIMIENTO: a canned roasted sweet red pepper; the mature pepper has its skin peeled off after roasting; a pimiento is softer than a roasted fresh red pepper.

POACH: to cook in water to cover at a temperature just lower than boiling, about 200°F.; a good method for all protein foods, as it does not toughen them.

POLYUNSATURATED: able to form many addition products in combination with other materials in the body; corn, soybean, safflower, sesame oils are examples; recommended for people on low-cholesterol diets. Cf. MONOUNSATURATED.

PROSCIUTTO: dry-cured raw Parma ham, dried in air-swept caves; delicate, delicious, flavorful; there is an American version.

PROVATURA: cheese made from buffalo's milk; like mozzarella, but made in smaller sizes; tender and juicy.

PURÉE: to reduce to a smooth homogeneous thick paste, in an electric blender, or by pushing through a food mill or sieve; esp. for fruits and vegetables.

RIB: see CELERY RIB and FENNEL RIB. The ribs of a pepper are inner membranes which are always trimmed away, as they are peppery.

RICOTTA: a smooth soft cheese, without curds, made from whey, with a rather sweet taste. American ricotta is made with milk.

RISOTTO: rice cooked with other ingredients.

RISTRETTI: reduced; used for clear soup concentrated to make it more flavorful. Cf. DOPPIO.

SAUTÉ: to cook in a small amount of oil over medium heat for a short time; the pan must be hot and the food must not be crowded.

SCALLOP: a small piece of boneless meat, a *scaloppina;* usually applied to a slice cut from the round of the veal leg.

SCALOPPINA, plural SCALOPPINE: see SCALLOP.

SCAMPO, plural SCAMPI: a lobsterette or langoustine, also called prawn, but not a shrimp; similar to a lobster in body shape; available frozen in U.S. markets.

SEAFOOD: fish, shellfish and crustaceans found in saltwater, used for food.

SHALLOT: an onion with a mild but intense flavor, which grows in a cluster of bulblets similarly to garlic. Each little bulb has a reddish or purple skin: before peeling one bulb may weigh about ¼ ounce.

SHELLFISH: a hard-shelled creature such as an oyster, clam or mussel. Although the shell of a squid is rudimentary, it is also a shellfish. Crustaceans are another kind of shellfish.

SHRED: to reduce to small pieces of random size and ragged shape; this can be done in a food grinder or an electric blender, or by hand with a chef's knife.

SIMMER: the same as poach as far as temperature is concerned, although it does not necessarily indicate that the food is covered with water.

SLURRY: a thin mixture of water and a starch (cornstarch, flour), which is added to other ingredients to thicken them.

SNIP: to reduce to small bits with a scissors; useful for chives and other herbs that are difficult to chop.

SOUFFLÉ: originally a baked dish, sweet or savory, containing beaten egg whites, which rose in the baking dish as air trapped in the beaten mixture expanded; later a cold dish piled up to resemble the baked dish and chilled, sometimes frozen. Cf. MOUSSE.

SPICE: a product of a tropical plant—the flower bud, seed, fleshy covering of the fruit, the root or tuber, bark, etc.; available whole (always preferred) and ground; most are dried, but some can be found fresh, e.g., gingerroot. Cf. HERB.

STEAM: to cook in steam rising from beneath the food; the liquid used can be water or stock. Cf. OIL-STEAM. Steaming is not recommended for leafy greens, as they will lose color.

STOCK: a liquid food made by extracting flavor and nutrients from various solid ingredients cooked in water for a long time; the basis of good soups and sauces, and useful as an ingredient in other recipes.

STRACCIATELLA: lit., rags; long thin strands of egg cooked in a broth, like Chinese "egg-drop soup."

STRAIN: to remove solid particles from a liquid; often the solid particles are discarded; the liquid is used. Cf. DRAIN. Stock that is strained is often treated further to remove minute particles. Cf. CLARIFY, 1.

TORTA: tart, pie, cake or pudding can all be called *torta;* it most nearly resembles a *quiche* in being baked in a shallow layer with no top, but a *torta* usually has no crust on the bottom either; a *torta* can be a first course, main course or dessert.

TORTINA: lit., a mini-*torta,* or tartlet, but usually a *tortina* is as large around as a *torta;* a *tortina* is an egg pie, made with vegetables, with or without a bottom crust of pastry or bread.

TOURNEDOS: a slice cut from the beef filet; usually about 1 inch thick, a tournedos weighs about 4 ounces. Cf. FILET MIGNON.

VEGETABLE OIL: an oil, liquid at room temperature, made from corn, cottonseed, peanut, safflower, sesame seed, soybean, etc.

VERDE: green; as in *salsa verde,* green sauce, indicating a sauce made from green herbs and vegetables.

VERDURE: green vegetables such as broccoli, escarole, spinach; leafy greens.

VITAMIN: an organic substance contained in foods, essential to the nutrition of humans; some are made in the body, but most need to be taken from food; vitamins regulate the body's metabolism.

ZABAGLIONE: a frothy mixture of eggs, or just egg yolks, with wine or liqueur and other flavoring; served as a dessert, hot, cold or frozen.

ZEST: the outermost layer of citrus rind, orange, lemon, lime, grapefruit, peeled off or grated off to use for flavoring.

ZUPPA: soup; used also for main-course "soups" with relatively little liquid, such as *zuppa di pesche.*

INDEX